# ~MemoryMinder~
## *Personal Health Journal*

## A Wellness Diary & Symptoms Log
### by MemoryMinder Journals

*"The ideal way to chronicle
health-related
habits and conditions"*

This journal belongs to

_____

From _____ To _____

**MemoryMinder** *Personal Health Journal*
Copyright ©1993, 1996 by F. & D. Wilkins
**MemoryMinder Journals, Inc.**
Printings: 1993, 1994, 1995, 1996,
Revised 1996, 1997, 1999, 2001
Revised 2003, 2004, 2005

**ISBN  0-9637968-0-1**
UPC 7-00703-81801-7

Illustrations from *Myofascial Pain and Dysfunction:
The Trigger Point Manual,* Volume 1
by Janet G. Travell, M.D. and David G. Simons, M.D.

For information regarding this publication, write to:
MemoryMinder Journals, Inc., P.O. Box 23108, Eugene, OR 97402-0425
www.memoryminder.com

**Printed and assembled in the USA**

## Do you ever...

...***wonder*** if there is a pattern to your health conditions?

...***wish*** you could remember exactly when certain conditions began or changed?

...***wish*** you could remember when you started taking a particular vitamin or medication?

...***wonder*** how much progress you have actually made toward your health goals?

...***wonder*** if the health regimen you are following is really making a difference in the way you feel?

...***forget*** to ask your doctor or other health-care provider an important question?

...***need*** to keep track of your health conditions for insurance or legal reasons?

...***feel*** too tired or too busy to write out all the little details that make up your health picture?

...***wish*** you had all your personal health information in a convenient and easy-to-retrieve format?

If you answered "yes" to any of these questions,
**MemoryMinder**
*Personal Health Journal*
is for you!

Other books by MemoryMinder Journals

•DietMinder
*Personal Food & Fitness Journal*

•BodyMinder
*Workout & Exercise Journal*

# ~Contents~

# ~Introduction~

If you have health concerns of any kind, the MemoryMinder Personal Health Journal can help you take control and become more aware of what *really* makes you tick!

Keeping track of the many factors that contribute to your health may seem to be an impossible task...but with this Journal you can record your conditions easily and quickly. The all-inclusive checklist format was designed to save time yet provide you with organized, consistent, easily retrievable, and *valuable* personal records.

Keeping a health diary can be beneficial in many ways; it's often an eye-opening experience! You may discover what has been causing a particular pain or other problem when you suddenly see the whole picture in black and white. You will be able to provide your doctor with much more complete and accurate information which is especially helpful if your condition is difficult to diagnose. If you spot habits that need improvement (such as diet or exercise) you'll be motivated to do better. After using your MemoryMinder for a while you'll see if the changes you've made in medications, vitamins, diet, etc. are really working.

Using a MemoryMinder can also be helpful for those who care for others (such as an elderly parent) who need care but are unable to handle the huge task of keeping everything straight. It gives the caregiver a secure feeling to be able to document details that might otherwise be forgotten.

We sincerely hope the MemoryMinder will bring you a new sense of control over your health. Some of the changes in this edition are the result of comments received from users of the original two versions. We appreciate those kind suggestions and, as before, welcome any new comments you may have.

# Tips for using
## *your*
# ~MemoryMinder~
## *Personal Health Journal*

Using your MemoryMinder is easy! The convenient checklist format is time-saving yet provides plenty of room for personalized record keeping. You don't have to use your Journal everyday-- it's entirely up to you. However, the more often you write in it, the more thorough and complete your records will be.

> Whether you use your Journal every day or just occasionally, a good rule of thumb to follow is:
> *Whenever your current health patterns or conditions change,* **record those changes.**

The following numbered paragraphs correspond to the sections in the illustration on the next page. Following these guidelines will assure you of receiving the maximum benefits from the use of your MemoryMinder.

**1** **Date** ... Be sure to fill in this box, and don't forget to include the day of the week. If you're required to take your blood pressure and sugar level readings each day, a place is provided to record this information along with your weight and body temperature. (For purposes of comparison, it is best if these readings are taken at the same time each day.) Your total hours of sleep (including naps) can also be recorded here.

**2** *Weather...* Over the years, many people have claimed that their health is affected by change in the weather. Sometimes just knowing that the weather may be the cause of certain pains, moods, or other responses can make them seem less worrisome. Check each box that applies to the day's weather.

**3** *Drugs/ Medications, Vitamins/ Herbs* ... Carefully complete these two areas. Include over-the-counter as well as prescription items, and don't forget to list the brand name and strength (500 mg., 400 i.u., etc.). Indicate the quantity and whether the substance was taken in the morning or the evening. Any injections you receive may be noted here as well. The information you record in this section might later prove to be an invaluable reference for you or your health-care provider.

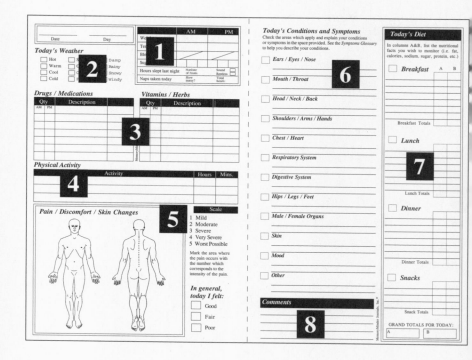

***Time-Saving Hint:*** After you have initially recorded your vitamin and medication data, you may want to simply write "same as usual" each day to save yourself time and effort. However, if you make *any changes* in your vitamins or medications, be sure that you make a new entry.

**4** ***Physical Activity . . .*** In addition to planned or specific exercises, be sure to include walks, gardening, vigorous housework, physical games, dancing, painting, moving, climbing stairs, etc.

**5** ***Pain / Discomfort . . .*** This is especially helpful for recording aches and pains that vary in intensity. On the illustrated figure, draw an arrow to the pain, then label it with the number corresponding to the intensity. You may also note what time of day the pain occurred. (See illustration.)

***Skin Changes . . .*** On the figure you can note any rashes, bites, bruises, or other skin conditions. You can also describe these conditions under "Skin" on the opposite page.

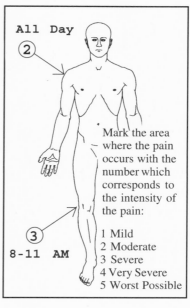

All Day
②

Mark the area where the pain occurs with the number which corresponds to the intensity of the pain:

1 Mild
2 Moderate
3 Severe
4 Very Severe
5 Worst Possible

③
8-11 AM

**6** ***Today's Conditions and Symptoms . . .*** Place a check mark beside any area where you have noticed a change or are having a problem. Then, in the space provided, briefly describe the specific problem. If needed, you may refer to the *Symptoms Glossary* following this section for help in describing your conditions.

**7** *Diet* . . . It's been said, *"You are what you eat."* It has also been said that many people have food allergies and don't even know it. Keeping a log of the foods you eat and drink may give you some new insight. If desired, you may record two types of nutritional data (i.e. fat, calories, sugar, sodium, carbohydrates, cholesterol, etc.) next to that particular food. At the bottom of this section, space is provided to list the applicable totals.

**8** *Comments* . . . Try to think of anything special about this day that could have some influence on your health. Briefly record any emotional feelings or experiences. Was it a stressful day? Did you visit your physician or dentist? Were you exposed to any contagious illnesses? Did you quit smoking? (Congratulations!) Did you use any new products, such as soaps, colognes, etc? These things may seem insignificant at the time, but may later be the key to understanding why you feel the way you do.

Sometimes it can be difficult to think of just the right word to describe a certain feeling or condition. For your convenience, a Symptoms Glossary has been provided following these Tips. This list is intended only to assist you in describing your conditions. It does not, of course, include all possible symptoms, and you may wish to use different wording to describe your particular condition.

*In the back of your Journal...* The colored pages in the last section of your MemoryMinder provide space for *Additional Health Records*. On these pages you can record your Personal Health History as well as Medical Tests. This data is especially handy when you visit a new doctor. In this section you may also record your Insurance & Pharmacy information and the names & addresses of your Health-Care Providers. You can keep track of health-related Purchases as well.

Most health-care advisors recommend taking a list of questions with you when you visit your doctor. This is a splendid idea! The MemoryMinder provides several pages for jotting down your <u>Notes & Questions</u>. If you write your questions down as soon as you think of them, you won't forget them, and it should make your health-care visit much more productive. (If you wish, you can skip a line or two between questions leaving space to write the answers you receive.)

There is a four-year reference calender following the Notes section and a reorder form in case MemoryMinders are not readily available at a store near you. Last but not least, in the back of the Journal, is a vinyl pocket-page. This is ideal for holding appointment cards, receipts, prescriptions, health articles, etc.

***Remember...*** Taking your MemoryMinder with you on visits to your doctor or other health-care provider will insure that you'll always have the information you need at your fingertips.

Best wishes for good health!

# ~Symptoms Glossary~

The following are descriptions of some conditions and symptoms which may apply to you. This list is intended only to assist you in describing your conditions. It does not, of course, include all possible symptoms. You may prefer to use different wording to describe your own particular conditions.

## Chest & Heart
Congestion
Heart flutters
Heart "pounds"
Pain
Tightness
Also see "Skin"

## Digestive System
*Appetite:*
Constant hunger
Excessive thirst
Food cravings
Poor appetite
*Bowels:*
Blood in stool
Constipation
Diarrhea
Excessive gas
Hemorrhoids
Irregularity
Rectal bleeding
Rectal pain/itching
Stools dark/light
*Urination:*
Blood in urine
Frequent
Infrequent
Painful
Poor bladder control

*Discomfort:*
Bloated
Burping
Heartburn
Hiccups
Indigestion
Intestinal pain
Nausea
Stomach ache
Vomiting

## Ears, Eyes & Nose
*Ears:*
Earache
Excessive Wax
Hearing Difficulty
Itching
Plugged
Ringing
*Eyes:*
Crusted lids
Dark circles
Discharge
Dry/Watery
Foreign object in
Itching, Irritated
Lids twitch
Red, Bloodshot
Sensitive to light
Swollen, Puffy
Vision blurry

*Nose:*
Bleeding
Congested
Dry
Itching
Runny, Discharge
Sinus pressure
Sore, Painful
Also see "Skin"

## Head, Neck & Back
Dandruff
Dizziness
Hair loss
Headache
 (mild/severe
 throbbing/dull
 stabbing/sinus- -
 denote location)
Itchy scalp
Lower back pain
Pain between
 shoulder blades
Stiffness
Also see "Skin"

## Hips, Legs & Feet
*Includes Knees, Ankles and Toes*
  Feet hot or cold
  Inflammation
  Joint pain
  Loss of feeling/Numb
  Muscle cramps
  Muscle pain
  Stiffness
  Swelling
  Tingling
  Also see "Skin"

## Male & Female Organs
*Male:*
  Discharge
  Impotence
  Infection
  Injury
  Itching
  Pain in genitals
  Rash or sores
*Female:*
  Breasts tender/swollen
  Breast lumps
  Discharge
  Genital itching
  Infection
  Menstrual cramps
  Period started/stopped
  Rash or sores
  Spotting
  Strong odor
  Vaginal dryness
  Also see "Skin"

## Mood
  Anxious
  Calm/Relaxed
  Confused
  Depressed
  Emotional
  Energetic
  Forgetful
  Irritable
  Listless
  Nervous
  Short-tempered
  Tense
  Unable to concentrate
  Worried

## Mouth & Throat
*Mouth:*
  Bad breath
  Bad taste
  Chapped lips
  Coated tongue
  Cold/Canker sores
  Dryness
  Gums sore/bleeding
  Jaw pain
  Sensitive teeth
  Sore tongue
  Toothache
*Throat:*
  Difficulty swallowing
  Frequent clearing
  Glands swollen
  Hoarseness, Laryngitis
  Red, Inflamed
  Sore

## Respiratory System
  Breathing irregular
  Congestion
  Coughing
  Hyper-ventilation
  Shortness of breath
  Sneezing
  Tight chest
  Wheezing

## Shoulders, Arms & Hands
*Includes Elbows, Wrists and Fingers*
  Fingernail changes
  Hands hot or cold
  Inflammation
  Joint pain
  Loss of feeling/Numb
  Muscle pain
  Stiffness
  Swelling
  Tingling
  Also see "Skin"

## Skin
  Bites
  Blemishes
  Chills, Goose Bumps
  Cold, Clammy
  Cuts, Bruises
  Dry, Flaky
  Excessive bleeding
  Flushed
  Heavy perspiration
  Hot flashes
  Hot, Feverish
  Itching
  Moles, new/changes
  Night sweats
  Numbness
  Rash
  Sunburn
  Swelling
  Tenderness
  Warts

## Other
  Excessive fatigue
  Fainting
  Insomnia
  Nightmares
  Overall weakness
  Shaking
  Water retention

*Daily  Record*
*of  your*
*Conditions  &  Habits*

| | AM | PM |
|---|---|---|
| Date _____ Day _____ | | |

## Today's Weather

- [ ] Hot
- [ ] Warm
- [ ] Cool
- [ ] Cold
- [ ] Sunny
- [ ] Cloudy
- [ ] Overcast
- [ ] Foggy
- [ ] Damp
- [ ] Rainy
- [ ] Snowy
- [ ] Windy

| | AM | PM |
|---|---|---|
| Weight | | |
| Temperature | | |
| Blood Pressure | | |
| Sugar Level | | |
| Hours slept last night | Number of hours: | Sound ☐ Restless ☐ |
| Naps taken today | How many? | Total hours: |

## Drugs / Medications

| Qty (AM / PM) | Description | Strength |
|---|---|---|
| | | |
| | | |
| | | |
| | | |
| | | |
| | | |
| | | |

## Vitamins / Herbs

| Qty (AM / PM) | Description | Strength |
|---|---|---|
| | | |
| | | |
| | | |
| | | |
| | | |
| | | |
| | | |

MemoryMinder©

## Physical Activity

| Activity | Hours | Mins. |
|---|---|---|
| | | |
| | | |
| | | |

## Pain / Discomfort / Skin Changes

**Scale**

1 Mild
2 Moderate
3 Severe
4 Very Severe
5 Worst Possible

Mark the area where the pain occurs with the number which corresponds to the intensity of the pain.

### In general, today I felt:

- [ ] Good
- [ ] Fair
- [ ] Poor

## Today's Conditions and Symptoms

Check the areas which apply and explain your conditions or symptoms in the space provided. See the *Symptoms Glossary* to help you describe your conditions.

☐ *Ears / Eyes / Nose*
_____

☐ *Mouth / Throat*
_____

☐ *Head / Neck / Back*
_____

☐ *Shoulders / Arms / Hands*
_____

☐ *Chest / Heart*
_____

☐ *Respiratory System*
_____

☐ *Digestive System*
_____

☐ *Hips / Legs / Feet*
_____

☐ *Male / Female Organs*
_____

☐ *Skin*
_____

☐ *Mood*
_____

☐ *Other*
_____
_____

## Comments
_____
_____
_____
_____

## Today's Diet

In columns A&B, list the nutritional facts you wish to monitor (i.e. fat, calories, sodium, sugar, protein, etc.)

| ☐ **Breakfast** | A | B |
|---|---|---|
|  |  |  |
|  |  |  |
|  |  |  |
|  |  |  |
|  |  |  |
| Breakfast Totals |  |  |

| ☐ **Lunch** |  |  |
|---|---|---|
|  |  |  |
|  |  |  |
|  |  |  |
|  |  |  |
|  |  |  |
| Lunch Totals |  |  |

| ☐ **Dinner** |  |  |
|---|---|---|
|  |  |  |
|  |  |  |
|  |  |  |
|  |  |  |
|  |  |  |
| Dinner Totals |  |  |

| ☐ **Snacks** |  |  |
|---|---|---|
|  |  |  |
|  |  |  |
|  |  |  |
| Snack Totals |  |  |

GRAND TOTALS FOR TODAY:

| A | B |
|---|---|
|  |  |

MemoryMinder©

_____ _____
Date                    Day

| | AM | PM |
|---|---|---|
| Weight | | |
| Temperature | | |
| Blood Pressure | | |
| Sugar Level | | |

## Today's Weather

- [ ] Hot
- [ ] Warm
- [ ] Cool
- [ ] Cold
- [ ] Sunny
- [ ] Cloudy
- [ ] Overcast
- [ ] Foggy
- [ ] Damp
- [ ] Rainy
- [ ] Snowy
- [ ] Windy

| | | |
|---|---|---|
| Hours slept last night | Number of hours: | Sound [ ] Restless [ ] |
| Naps taken today | How many? | Total hours: |

## Drugs / Medications

| Qty | | Description | Strength |
|---|---|---|---|
| AM | PM | | |
| | | | |
| | | | |
| | | | |
| | | | |
| | | | |
| | | | |
| | | | |

## Vitamins / Herbs

| Qty | | Description | Strengt |
|---|---|---|---|
| AM | PM | | |
| | | | |
| | | | |
| | | | |
| | | | |
| | | | |
| | | | |
| | | | |

MemoryMinder©

## Physical Activity

| Activity | Hours | Mins. |
|---|---|---|
| | | |
| | | |
| | | |

## Pain / Discomfort / Skin Changes

### Scale

1 Mild
2 Moderate
3 Severe
4 Very Severe
5 Worst Possible

Mark the area where the pain occurs with the number which corresponds to the intensity of the pain.

### In general, today I felt:

- [ ] Good
- [ ] Fair
- [ ] Poor

## Today's Conditions and Symptoms

Check the areas which apply and explain your conditions or symptoms in the space provided. See the *Symptoms Glossary* to help you describe your conditions.

☐ *Ears / Eyes / Nose*

_____

☐ *Mouth / Throat*

_____

☐ *Head / Neck / Back*

_____

☐ *Shoulders / Arms / Hands*

_____

☐ *Chest / Heart*

_____

☐ *Respiratory System*

_____

☐ *Digestive System*

_____

☐ *Hips / Legs / Feet*

_____

☐ *Male / Female Organs*

_____

☐ *Skin*

_____

☐ *Mood*

_____

☐ *Other*

_____
_____

## Comments

_____
_____
_____
_____

## Today's Diet

In columns A&B, list the nutritional facts you wish to monitor (i.e. fat, calories, sodium, sugar, protein, etc.)

| ☐ **Breakfast** | A | B |
|---|---|---|
| | | |
| | | |
| | | |
| | | |
| | | |
| Breakfast Totals | | |

| ☐ **Lunch** | | |
|---|---|---|
| | | |
| | | |
| | | |
| | | |
| | | |
| Lunch Totals | | |

| ☐ **Dinner** | | |
|---|---|---|
| | | |
| | | |
| | | |
| | | |
| | | |
| Dinner Totals | | |

| ☐ **Snacks** | | |
|---|---|---|
| | | |
| | | |
| | | |
| Snack Totals | | |

| GRAND TOTALS FOR TODAY: | |
|---|---|
| A | B |
| | |

MemoryMinder©

| | Date | | Day |
|---|---|---|---|

|  | AM | PM |
|---|---|---|
| Weight | | |
| Temperature | | |
| Blood Pressure | | |
| Sugar Level | | |
| Hours slept last night | Number of hours: | Sound ☐ Restless ☐ |
| Naps taken today | How many? | Total hours: |

## Today's Weather

☐ Hot    ☐ Sunny    ☐ Damp
☐ Warm    ☐ Cloudy    ☐ Rainy
☐ Cool    ☐ Overcast    ☐ Snowy
☐ Cold    ☐ Foggy    ☐ Windy

## Drugs / Medications

| Qty | | Description | Strength |
|---|---|---|---|
| AM | PM | | |
| | | | |
| | | | |
| | | | |
| | | | |
| | | | |
| | | | |

## Vitamins / Herbs

| Qty | | Description | Strength |
|---|---|---|---|
| AM | PM | | |
| | | | |
| | | | |
| | | | |
| | | | |
| | | | |
| | | | |

MemoryMinder©

## Physical Activity

| Activity | Hours | Mins. |
|---|---|---|
| | | |
| | | |
| | | |
| | | |

## Pain / Discomfort / Skin Changes

### Scale

1 Mild
2 Moderate
3 Severe
4 Very Severe
5 Worst Possible

Mark the area where the pain occurs with the number which corresponds to the intensity of the pain.

### In general, today I felt:

☐ Good
☐ Fair
☐ Poor

## Today's Conditions and Symptoms

Check the areas which apply and explain your conditions or symptoms in the space provided. See the *Symptoms Glossary* to help you describe your conditions.

☐ *Ears / Eyes / Nose*
_____

☐ *Mouth / Throat*
_____

☐ *Head / Neck / Back*
_____

☐ *Shoulders / Arms / Hands*
_____

☐ *Chest / Heart*
_____

☐ *Respiratory System*
_____

☐ *Digestive System*
_____

☐ *Hips / Legs / Feet*
_____

☐ *Male / Female Organs*
_____

☐ *Skin*
_____

☐ *Mood*
_____

☐ *Other*
_____

## Comments
_____
_____
_____
_____

MemoryMinder©

## Today's Diet

In columns A&B, list the nutritional facts you wish to monitor (i.e. fat, calories, sodium, sugar, protein, etc.)

| ☐ **Breakfast** | A | B |
|---|---|---|
| | | |
| | | |
| | | |
| | | |
| | | |
| Breakfast Totals | | |

| ☐ **Lunch** | | |
|---|---|---|
| | | |
| | | |
| | | |
| | | |
| | | |
| Lunch Totals | | |

| ☐ **Dinner** | | |
|---|---|---|
| | | |
| | | |
| | | |
| | | |
| | | |
| Dinner Totals | | |

| ☐ **Snacks** | | |
|---|---|---|
| | | |
| | | |
| Snack Totals | | |

GRAND TOTALS FOR TODAY:

| A | B |
|---|---|
| | |

| | _____ | _____ |
|---|---|---|
| | Date | Day |

| | | AM | PM |
|---|---|---|---|
| Weight | | | |
| Temperature | | | |
| Blood Pressure | | | |
| Sugar Level | | | |
| Hours slept last night | | Number of hours: | Sound ☐ Restless ☐ |
| Naps taken today | | How many? | Total hours: |

## Today's Weather

☐ Hot    ☐ Sunny    ☐ Damp
☐ Warm    ☐ Cloudy    ☐ Rainy
☐ Cool    ☐ Overcast    ☐ Snowy
☐ Cold    ☐ Foggy    ☐ Windy

## Drugs / Medications

| Qty | | Description | Strength |
|---|---|---|---|
| AM | PM | | |
| | | | |
| | | | |
| | | | |
| | | | |
| | | | |
| | | | |

## Vitamins / Herbs

| Qty | | Description | Strength |
|---|---|---|---|
| AM | PM | | |
| | | | |
| | | | |
| | | | |
| | | | |
| | | | |

MemoryMinder©

## Physical Activity

| Activity | Hours | Mins. |
|---|---|---|
| | | |
| | | |
| | | |

## Pain / Discomfort / Skin Changes

### Scale

1 Mild
2 Moderate
3 Severe
4 Very Severe
5 Worst Possible

Mark the area where the pain occurs with the number which corresponds to the intensity of the pain.

### In general, today I felt:

☐ Good
☐ Fair
☐ Poor

## Today's Conditions and Symptoms

Check the areas which apply and explain your conditions or symptoms in the space provided. See the *Symptoms Glossary* to help you describe your conditions.

☐ *Ears / Eyes / Nose*
_____
_____

☐ *Mouth / Throat*
_____
_____

☐ *Head / Neck / Back*
_____
_____

☐ *Shoulders / Arms / Hands*
_____
_____

☐ *Chest / Heart*
_____
_____

☐ *Respiratory System*
_____
_____

☐ *Digestive System*
_____
_____

☐ *Hips / Legs / Feet*
_____
_____

☐ *Male / Female Organs*
_____
_____

☐ *Skin*
_____
_____

☐ *Mood*
_____
_____

☐ *Other*
_____
_____
_____

## Comments
_____
_____
_____
_____
_____

## Today's Diet

In columns A&B, list the nutritional facts you wish to monitor (i.e. fat, calories, sodium, sugar, protein, etc.)

☐ **Breakfast**    A    B

Breakfast Totals

☐ **Lunch**

Lunch Totals

☐ **Dinner**

Dinner Totals

☐ **Snacks**

Snack Totals

GRAND TOTALS FOR TODAY:

| A | B |
|---|---|
|   |   |

MemoryMinder©

| | Date | | Day | |
|---|---|---|---|---|

|  | AM | PM |
|---|---|---|
| Weight | | |
| Temperature | | |
| Blood Pressure | | |
| Sugar Level | | |
| Hours slept last night | Number of hours: | Sound ☐ Restless ☐ |
| Naps taken today | How many? | Total hours: |

## Today's Weather

- ☐ Hot
- ☐ Warm
- ☐ Cool
- ☐ Cold
- ☐ Sunny
- ☐ Cloudy
- ☐ Overcast
- ☐ Foggy
- ☐ Damp
- ☐ Rainy
- ☐ Snowy
- ☐ Windy

## Drugs / Medications

| Qty | | Description | Strength |
|---|---|---|---|
| AM | PM | | |
| | | | |
| | | | |
| | | | |
| | | | |
| | | | |
| | | | |

## Vitamins / Herbs

| Qty | | Description | Strength |
|---|---|---|---|
| AM | PM | | |
| | | | |
| | | | |
| | | | |
| | | | |
| | | | |
| | | | |

MemoryMinder©

## Physical Activity

| Activity | Hours | Mins. |
|---|---|---|
| | | |
| | | |
| | | |

## Pain / Discomfort / Skin Changes

### Scale

1 Mild
2 Moderate
3 Severe
4 Very Severe
5 Worst Possible

Mark the area where the pain occurs with the number which corresponds to the intensity of the pain.

### In general, today I felt:

- ☐ Good
- ☐ Fair
- ☐ Poor

## Today's Conditions and Symptoms

Check the areas which apply and explain your conditions or symptoms in the space provided. See the *Symptoms Glossary* to help you describe your conditions.

☐ *Ears / Eyes / Nose*

_____

☐ *Mouth / Throat*

_____

☐ *Head / Neck / Back*

_____

☐ *Shoulders / Arms / Hands*

_____

☐ *Chest / Heart*

_____

☐ *Respiratory System*

_____

☐ *Digestive System*

_____

☐ *Hips / Legs / Feet*

_____

☐ *Male / Female Organs*

_____

☐ *Skin*

_____

☐ *Mood*

_____

☐ *Other*

_____

## Comments

_____
_____
_____
_____

MemoryMinder©

## Today's Diet

In columns A&B, list the nutritional facts you wish to monitor (i.e. fat, calories, sodium, sugar, protein, etc.)

| ☐ **Breakfast** | A | B |
|---|---|---|
| | | |
| | | |
| | | |
| | | |
| Breakfast Totals | | |

| ☐ **Lunch** | | |
|---|---|---|
| | | |
| | | |
| | | |
| | | |
| | | |
| Lunch Totals | | |

| ☐ **Dinner** | | |
|---|---|---|
| | | |
| | | |
| | | |
| | | |
| | | |
| Dinner Totals | | |

| ☐ **Snacks** | | |
|---|---|---|
| | | |
| | | |
| | | |
| Snack Totals | | |

GRAND TOTALS FOR TODAY:

| A | B |
|---|---|
| | |

|  | Date |  | Day |
|---|---|---|---|

| | AM | PM |
|---|---|---|
| Weight | | |
| Temperature | | |
| Blood Pressure | | |
| Sugar Level | | |
| Hours slept last night | Number of hours: | Sound ☐ Restless ☐ |
| Naps taken today | How many? | Total hours: |

## Today's Weather

☐ Hot    ☐ Sunny    ☐ Damp
☐ Warm    ☐ Cloudy    ☐ Rainy
☐ Cool    ☐ Overcast    ☐ Snowy
☐ Cold    ☐ Foggy    ☐ Windy

## Drugs / Medications

| Qty | | Description | Strength |
|---|---|---|---|
| AM | PM | | |
| | | | |
| | | | |
| | | | |
| | | | |
| | | | |
| | | | |

## Vitamins / Herbs

| Qty | | Description | Strength |
|---|---|---|---|
| AM | PM | | |
| | | | |
| | | | |
| | | | |
| | | | |
| | | | |
| | | | |

MemoryMinder©

## Physical Activity

| Activity | Hours | Mins. |
|---|---|---|
| | | |
| | | |
| | | |

## Pain / Discomfort / Skin Changes

### Scale

1 Mild
2 Moderate
3 Severe
4 Very Severe
5 Worst Possible

Mark the area where the pain occurs with the number which corresponds to the intensity of the pain.

### In general, today I felt:

☐ Good
☐ Fair
☐ Poor

## Today's Conditions and Symptoms

Check the areas which apply and explain your conditions or symptoms in the space provided. See the *Symptoms Glossary* to help you describe your conditions.

☐ *Ears / Eyes / Nose*

_____

☐ *Mouth / Throat*

_____

☐ *Head / Neck / Back*

_____

☐ *Shoulders / Arms / Hands*

_____

☐ *Chest / Heart*

_____

☐ *Respiratory System*

_____

☐ *Digestive System*

_____

☐ *Hips / Legs / Feet*

_____

☐ *Male / Female Organs*

_____

☐ *Skin*

_____

☐ *Mood*

_____

☐ *Other*

_____
_____

## Comments

_____
_____
_____
_____

MemoryMinder©

## Today's Diet

In columns A&B, list the nutritional facts you wish to monitor (i.e. fat, calories, sodium, sugar, protein, etc.)

☐ *Breakfast*

| | A | B |
|---|---|---|
| | | |
| | | |
| | | |
| | | |
| Breakfast Totals | | |

☐ *Lunch*

| | A | B |
|---|---|---|
| | | |
| | | |
| | | |
| | | |
| Lunch Totals | | |

☐ *Dinner*

| | A | B |
|---|---|---|
| | | |
| | | |
| | | |
| | | |
| Dinner Totals | | |

☐ *Snacks*

| | A | B |
|---|---|---|
| | | |
| | | |
| Snack Totals | | |

GRAND TOTALS FOR TODAY:

| A | B |
|---|---|
| | |

| | | Date | | | Day | |
|---|---|---|---|---|---|---|

## Today's Weather

- [ ] Hot
- [ ] Warm
- [ ] Cool
- [ ] Cold
- [ ] Sunny
- [ ] Cloudy
- [ ] Overcast
- [ ] Foggy
- [ ] Damp
- [ ] Rainy
- [ ] Snowy
- [ ] Windy

| | AM | PM |
|---|---|---|
| Weight | | |
| Temperature | | |
| Blood Pressure | | |
| Sugar Level | | |
| Hours slept last night | Number of hours: | Sound ☐ Restless ☐ |
| Naps taken today | How many? | Total hours: |

## Drugs / Medications

| Qty | | Description | Strength |
|---|---|---|---|
| AM | PM | | |
| | | | |
| | | | |
| | | | |
| | | | |
| | | | |
| | | | |

## Vitamins / Herbs

| Qty | | Description | Strength |
|---|---|---|---|
| AM | PM | | |
| | | | |
| | | | |
| | | | |
| | | | |
| | | | |
| | | | |

MemoryMinder©

## Physical Activity

| Activity | Hours | Mins |
|---|---|---|
| | | |
| | | |
| | | |

## Pain / Discomfort / Skin Changes

### Scale

1 Mild
2 Moderate
3 Severe
4 Very Severe
5 Worst Possible

Mark the area where the pain occurs with the number which corresponds to the intensity of the pain.

### In general, today I felt:

- [ ] Good
- [ ] Fair
- [ ] Poor

## Today's Conditions and Symptoms

Check the areas which apply and explain your conditions or symptoms in the space provided. See the *Symptoms Glossary* to help you describe your conditions.

☐ *Ears / Eyes / Nose*

_____

☐ *Mouth / Throat*

_____

☐ *Head / Neck / Back*

_____

☐ *Shoulders / Arms / Hands*

_____

☐ *Chest / Heart*

_____

☐ *Respiratory System*

_____

☐ *Digestive System*

_____

☐ *Hips / Legs / Feet*

_____

☐ *Male / Female Organs*

_____

☐ *Skin*

_____

☐ *Mood*

_____

☐ *Other*

_____
_____

## Comments

_____
_____
_____
_____

MemoryMinder©

## Today's Diet

In columns A&B, list the nutritional facts you wish to monitor (i.e. fat, calories, sodium, sugar, protein, etc.)

☐ **Breakfast**   A   B

Breakfast Totals

☐ **Lunch**

Lunch Totals

☐ **Dinner**

Dinner Totals

☐ **Snacks**

Snack Totals

GRAND TOTALS FOR TODAY:

A _____   B _____

| | Date | | Day | |
|---|---|---|---|---|

## Today's Weather

- [ ] Hot
- [ ] Warm
- [ ] Cool
- [ ] Cold
- [ ] Sunny
- [ ] Cloudy
- [ ] Overcast
- [ ] Foggy
- [ ] Damp
- [ ] Rainy
- [ ] Snowy
- [ ] Windy

| | AM | PM |
|---|---|---|
| Weight | | |
| Temperature | | |
| Blood Pressure | | |
| Sugar Level | | |
| Hours slept last night | Number of hours: | Sound ☐ Restless ☐ |
| Naps taken today | How many? | Total hours: |

## Drugs / Medications

| Qty | | Description | Strength |
|---|---|---|---|
| AM | PM | | |
| | | | |
| | | | |
| | | | |
| | | | |
| | | | |
| | | | |

## Vitamins / Herbs

| Qty | | Description | Strengt |
|---|---|---|---|
| AM | PM | | |
| | | | |
| | | | |
| | | | |
| | | | |
| | | | |
| | | | |

MemoryMinder©

## Physical Activity

| Activity | Hours | Mins |
|---|---|---|
| | | |
| | | |
| | | |

## Pain / Discomfort / Skin Changes

### Scale

1 Mild
2 Moderate
3 Severe
4 Very Severe
5 Worst Possible

Mark the area where the pain occurs with the number which corresponds to the intensity of the pain.

### In general, today I felt:

- [ ] Good
- [ ] Fair
- [ ] Poor

# Today's Conditions and Symptoms

Check the areas which apply and explain your conditions or symptoms in the space provided. See the *Symptoms Glossary* to help you describe your conditions.

☐ *Ears / Eyes / Nose*
_____
_____

☐ *Mouth / Throat*
_____
_____

☐ *Head / Neck / Back*
_____
_____

☐ *Shoulders / Arms / Hands*
_____
_____

☐ *Chest / Heart*
_____
_____

☐ *Respiratory System*
_____
_____

☐ *Digestive System*
_____
_____

☐ *Hips / Legs / Feet*
_____
_____

☐ *Male / Female Organs*
_____
_____

☐ *Skin*
_____
_____

☐ *Mood*
_____
_____

☐ *Other*
_____
_____
_____

## Comments
_____
_____
_____
_____

MemoryMinder©

# Today's Diet

In columns A&B, list the nutritional facts you wish to monitor (i.e. fat, calories, sodium, sugar, protein, etc.)

| ☐ **Breakfast** | A | B |
|---|---|---|
| | | |
| | | |
| | | |
| | | |
| | | |
| Breakfast Totals | | |

| ☐ **Lunch** | | |
|---|---|---|
| | | |
| | | |
| | | |
| | | |
| | | |
| Lunch Totals | | |

| ☐ **Dinner** | | |
|---|---|---|
| | | |
| | | |
| | | |
| | | |
| | | |
| | | |
| Dinner Totals | | |

| ☐ **Snacks** | | |
|---|---|---|
| | | |
| | | |
| | | |
| Snack Totals | | |

GRAND TOTALS FOR TODAY:

| A | B |
|---|---|
| | |

| _____ _____ | | AM | PM |
|---|---|---|---|
| Date          Day | Weight | | |
| | Temperature | | |
| **Today's Weather** | Blood Pressure | / | / |
| | Sugar Level | | |
| | Hours slept last night | Number of hours: | Sound / Restless |
| | Naps taken today | How many? | Total hours: |

**Today's Weather**

- [ ] Hot
- [ ] Warm
- [ ] Cool
- [ ] Cold
- [ ] Sunny
- [ ] Cloudy
- [ ] Overcast
- [ ] Foggy
- [ ] Damp
- [ ] Rainy
- [ ] Snowy
- [ ] Windy

## Drugs / Medications

| Qty | | Description | Strength |
|---|---|---|---|
| AM | PM | | |
| | | | |
| | | | |
| | | | |
| | | | |
| | | | |
| | | | |

## Vitamins / Herbs

| Qty | | Description | Strength |
|---|---|---|---|
| AM | PM | | |
| | | | |
| | | | |
| | | | |
| | | | |
| | | | |

MemoryMinder©

## Physical Activity

| Activity | Hours | Mins. |
|---|---|---|
| | | |
| | | |
| | | |

## Pain / Discomfort / Skin Changes

### Scale

1 Mild
2 Moderate
3 Severe
4 Very Severe
5 Worst Possible

Mark the area where the pain occurs with the number which corresponds to the intensity of the pain.

### In general, today I felt:

- [ ] Good
- [ ] Fair
- [ ] Poor

## Today's Conditions and Symptoms

Check the areas which apply and explain your conditions or symptoms in the space provided. See the *Symptoms Glossary* to help you describe your conditions.

☐ *Ears / Eyes / Nose*
_____
_____

☐ *Mouth / Throat*
_____
_____

☐ *Head / Neck / Back*
_____
_____

☐ *Shoulders / Arms / Hands*
_____
_____

☐ *Chest / Heart*
_____
_____

☐ *Respiratory System*
_____
_____

☐ *Digestive System*
_____
_____

☐ *Hips / Legs / Feet*
_____
_____

☐ *Male / Female Organs*
_____
_____

☐ *Skin*
_____
_____

☐ *Mood*
_____
_____

☐ *Other*
_____
_____
_____

## Comments
_____
_____
_____
_____

## Today's Diet

In columns A&B, list the nutritional facts you wish to monitor (i.e. fat, calories, sodium, sugar, protein, etc.)

| ☐ *Breakfast* | A | B |
|---|---|---|
|  |  |  |
|  |  |  |
|  |  |  |
|  |  |  |
|  |  |  |
| Breakfast Totals |  |  |

| ☐ *Lunch* |  |  |
|---|---|---|
|  |  |  |
|  |  |  |
|  |  |  |
|  |  |  |
|  |  |  |
| Lunch Totals |  |  |

| ☐ *Dinner* |  |  |
|---|---|---|
|  |  |  |
|  |  |  |
|  |  |  |
|  |  |  |
|  |  |  |
| Dinner Totals |  |  |

| ☐ *Snacks* |  |  |
|---|---|---|
|  |  |  |
|  |  |  |
|  |  |  |
| Snack Totals |  |  |

GRAND TOTALS FOR TODAY:

| A | B |
|---|---|
|  |  |

MemoryMinder©

| | | AM | PM |
|---|---|---|---|
| _____ _____ | Weight | | |
| Date       Day | Temperature | | |
| | Blood Pressure | | |
| | Sugar Level | | |
| | Hours slept last night | Number of hours: | Sound ☐ Restless ☐ |
| | Naps taken today | How many? | Total hours: |

## Today's Weather

☐ Hot      ☐ Sunny      ☐ Damp
☐ Warm     ☐ Cloudy     ☐ Rainy
☐ Cool     ☐ Overcast   ☐ Snowy
☐ Cold     ☐ Foggy      ☐ Windy

## Drugs / Medications

| Qty | | Description | Strength |
|---|---|---|---|
| AM | PM | | |
| | | | |
| | | | |
| | | | |
| | | | |
| | | | |
| | | | |

## Vitamins / Herbs

| Qty | | Description | Strengt |
|---|---|---|---|
| AM | PM | | |
| | | | |
| | | | |
| | | | |
| | | | |
| | | | |
| | | | |

MemoryMinder©

## Physical Activity

| Activity | Hours | Mins |
|---|---|---|
| | | |
| | | |
| | | |

## Pain / Discomfort / Skin Changes

### Scale

1 Mild
2 Moderate
3 Severe
4 Very Severe
5 Worst Possible

Mark the area where the pain occurs with the number which corresponds to the intensity of the pain.

### In general, today I felt:

☐ Good
☐ Fair
☐ Poor

## Today's Conditions and Symptoms

Check the areas which apply and explain your conditions or symptoms in the space provided. See the *Symptoms Glossary* to help you describe your conditions.

☐ *Ears / Eyes / Nose*
_____

☐ *Mouth / Throat*
_____

☐ *Head / Neck / Back*
_____

☐ *Shoulders / Arms / Hands*
_____

☐ *Chest / Heart*
_____

☐ *Respiratory System*
_____

☐ *Digestive System*
_____

☐ *Hips / Legs / Feet*
_____

☐ *Male / Female Organs*
_____

☐ *Skin*
_____

☐ *Mood*
_____

☐ *Other*
_____
_____

## Comments
_____
_____
_____
_____

## Today's Diet

In columns A&B, list the nutritional facts you wish to monitor (i.e. fat, calories, sodium, sugar, protein, etc.)

| ☐ *Breakfast* | A | B |
|---|---|---|
| | | |
| | | |
| | | |
| | | |
| Breakfast Totals | | |

| ☐ *Lunch* | | |
|---|---|---|
| | | |
| | | |
| | | |
| | | |
| Lunch Totals | | |

| ☐ *Dinner* | | |
|---|---|---|
| | | |
| | | |
| | | |
| | | |
| | | |
| Dinner Totals | | |

| ☐ *Snacks* | | |
|---|---|---|
| | | |
| | | |
| | | |
| Snack Totals | | |

GRAND TOTALS FOR TODAY:

| A | B |
|---|---|
| | |

MemoryMinder©

_____   _____
Date                    Day

| | AM | PM |
|---|---|---|
| Weight | | |
| Temperature | | |
| Blood Pressure | | |
| Sugar Level | | |

## Today's Weather

- [ ] Hot
- [ ] Warm
- [ ] Cool
- [ ] Cold
- [ ] Sunny
- [ ] Cloudy
- [ ] Overcast
- [ ] Foggy
- [ ] Damp
- [ ] Rainy
- [ ] Snowy
- [ ] Windy

| Hours slept last night | Number of hours: | Sound [ ] Restless [ ] |
|---|---|---|
| Naps taken today | How many? | Total hours: |

## Drugs / Medications

| Qty | | Description | Strength |
|---|---|---|---|
| AM | PM | | |
| | | | |
| | | | |
| | | | |
| | | | |
| | | | |
| | | | |

MemoryMinder©

## Vitamins / Herbs

| Qty | | Description | Strengt |
|---|---|---|---|
| AM | PM | | |
| | | | |
| | | | |
| | | | |
| | | | |
| | | | |
| | | | |

## Physical Activity

| Activity | Hours | Mins. |
|---|---|---|
| | | |
| | | |
| | | |

## Pain / Discomfort / Skin Changes

### Scale

1 Mild
2 Moderate
3 Severe
4 Very Severe
5 Worst Possible

Mark the area where the pain occurs with the number which corresponds to the intensity of the pain.

### In general, today I felt:

- [ ] Good
- [ ] Fair
- [ ] Poor

# Today's Conditions and Symptoms

Check the areas which apply and explain your conditions or symptoms in the space provided. See the *Symptoms Glossary* to help you describe your conditions.

☐ **Ears / Eyes / Nose**

_____

☐ **Mouth / Throat**

_____

☐ **Head / Neck / Back**

_____

☐ **Shoulders / Arms / Hands**

_____

☐ **Chest / Heart**

_____

☐ **Respiratory System**

_____

☐ **Digestive System**

_____

☐ **Hips / Legs / Feet**

_____

☐ **Male / Female Organs**

_____

☐ **Skin**

_____

☐ **Mood**

_____

☐ **Other**

_____
_____

# Comments

_____
_____
_____
_____

MemoryMinder©

# Today's Diet

In columns A&B, list the nutritional facts you wish to monitor (i.e. fat, calories, sodium, sugar, protein, etc.)

| ☐ **Breakfast** | A | B |
|---|---|---|
| | | |
| | | |
| | | |
| | | |
| | | |
| Breakfast Totals | | |

| ☐ **Lunch** | | |
|---|---|---|
| | | |
| | | |
| | | |
| | | |
| | | |
| Lunch Totals | | |

| ☐ **Dinner** | | |
|---|---|---|
| | | |
| | | |
| | | |
| | | |
| | | |
| Dinner Totals | | |

| ☐ **Snacks** | | |
|---|---|---|
| | | |
| | | |
| | | |
| Snack Totals | | |

GRAND TOTALS FOR TODAY:

| A | B |
|---|---|
| | |

| _____ _____ | | AM | PM |
|---|---|---|---|
| Date / Day | Weight | | |
| | Temperature | | |

## Today's Weather

| | AM | PM |
|---|---|---|
| Weight | | |
| Temperature | | |
| Blood Pressure | | |
| Sugar Level | | |

- ☐ Hot
- ☐ Warm
- ☐ Cool
- ☐ Cold
- ☐ Sunny
- ☐ Cloudy
- ☐ Overcast
- ☐ Foggy
- ☐ Damp
- ☐ Rainy
- ☐ Snowy
- ☐ Windy

| Hours slept last night | Number of hours: | Sound ☐ Restless ☐ |
| Naps taken today | How many? | Total hours: |

## Drugs / Medications

| Qty | | Description | Strength |
|---|---|---|---|
| AM | PM | | |
| | | | |
| | | | |
| | | | |
| | | | |
| | | | |
| | | | |
| | | | |

## Vitamins / Herbs

| Qty | | Description | Strength |
|---|---|---|---|
| AM | PM | | |
| | | | |
| | | | |
| | | | |
| | | | |
| | | | |
| | | | |

MemoryMinder©

## Physical Activity

| Activity | Hours | Mins. |
|---|---|---|
| | | |
| | | |
| | | |

## Pain / Discomfort / Skin Changes

### Scale

1 Mild
2 Moderate
3 Severe
4 Very Severe
5 Worst Possible

Mark the area where the pain occurs with the number which corresponds to the intensity of the pain.

### In general, today I felt:

- ☐ Good
- ☐ Fair
- ☐ Poor

# Today's Conditions and Symptoms

Check the areas which apply and explain your conditions & symptoms in the space provided. See the *Symptoms glossary* to help you describe your conditions.

☐ *Ears / Eyes / Nose*
_____
_____

☐ *Mouth / Throat*
_____
_____

☐ *Head / Neck / Back*
_____
_____

☐ *Shoulders / Arms / Hands*
_____
_____

☐ *Chest / Heart*
_____
_____

☐ *Respiratory System*
_____
_____

☐ *Digestive System*
_____
_____

☐ *Hips / Legs / Feet*
_____
_____

☐ *Male / Female Organs*
_____
_____

☐ *Skin*
_____
_____

☐ *Mood*
_____
_____

☐ *Other*
_____
_____

## Comments
_____
_____
_____
_____

## Today's Diet

In columns A&B, list the nutritional facts you wish to monitor (i.e. fat, calories, sodium, sugar, protein, etc.)

☐ **Breakfast**    A    B

Breakfast Totals

☐ **Lunch**

Lunch Totals

☐ **Dinner**

Dinner Totals

☐ **Snacks**

Snack Totals

GRAND TOTALS FOR TODAY:

A _____    B _____

MemoryMinder©

| | Date | | Day |
| --- | --- | --- | --- |

| | | AM | PM |
| --- | --- | --- | --- |
| Weight | | | |
| Temperature | | | |
| Blood Pressure | | | |
| Sugar Level | | | |
| Hours slept last night | Number of hours: | | Sound ☐ Restless ☐ |
| Naps taken today | How many? | | Total hours: |

## Today's Weather

- ☐ Hot
- ☐ Warm
- ☐ Cool
- ☐ Cold
- ☐ Sunny
- ☐ Cloudy
- ☐ Overcast
- ☐ Foggy
- ☐ Damp
- ☐ Rainy
- ☐ Snowy
- ☐ Windy

## Drugs / Medications

| Qty | | Description | Strength |
| --- | --- | --- | --- |
| AM | PM | | |
| | | | |
| | | | |
| | | | |
| | | | |
| | | | |
| | | | |

## Vitamins / Herbs

| Qty | | Description | Strengt |
| --- | --- | --- | --- |
| AM | PM | | |
| | | | |
| | | | |
| | | | |
| | | | |
| | | | |

MemoryMinder©

## Physical Activity

| Activity | Hours | Mins. |
| --- | --- | --- |
| | | |
| | | |
| | | |

## Pain / Discomfort / Skin Changes

### Scale

1 Mild
2 Moderate
3 Severe
4 Very Severe
5 Worst Possible

Mark the area where the pain occurs with the number which corresponds to the intensity of the pain.

### In general, today I felt:

- ☐ Good
- ☐ Fair
- ☐ Poor

## Today's Conditions and Symptoms

Check the areas which apply and explain your conditions or symptoms in the space provided. See the *Symptoms Glossary* to help you describe your conditions.

☐ *Ears / Eyes / Nose*
_____
_____

☐ *Mouth / Throat*
_____
_____

☐ *Head / Neck / Back*
_____
_____

☐ *Shoulders / Arms / Hands*
_____
_____

☐ *Chest / Heart*
_____
_____

☐ *Respiratory System*
_____
_____

☐ *Digestive System*
_____
_____

☐ *Hips / Legs / Feet*
_____
_____

☐ *Male / Female Organs*
_____
_____

☐ *Skin*
_____
_____

☐ *Mood*
_____
_____

☐ *Other*
_____
_____

## Comments
_____
_____
_____
_____

## Today's Diet

In columns A&B, list the nutritional facts you wish to monitor (i.e. fat, calories, sodium, sugar, protein, etc.)

| ☐ **Breakfast** | A | B |
|---|---|---|
| | | |
| | | |
| | | |
| | | |
| | | |
| Breakfast Totals | | |

| ☐ **Lunch** | | |
|---|---|---|
| | | |
| | | |
| | | |
| | | |
| | | |
| Lunch Totals | | |

| ☐ **Dinner** | | |
|---|---|---|
| | | |
| | | |
| | | |
| | | |
| | | |
| Dinner Totals | | |

| ☐ **Snacks** | | |
|---|---|---|
| | | |
| | | |
| | | |
| Snack Totals | | |

GRAND TOTALS FOR TODAY:

| A | B |
|---|---|
| . | |

MemoryMinder©

| | | AM | PM |
|---|---|---|---|
| Date _____ Day _____ | Weight | | |
| | Temperature | | |
| | Blood Pressure | | |
| | Sugar Level | | | | |
| | Hours slept last night | Number of hours: | Sound ☐ Restless ☐ |
| | Naps taken today | How many? | Total hours: |

## Today's Weather

☐ Hot        ☐ Sunny        ☐ Damp
☐ Warm       ☐ Cloudy       ☐ Rainy
☐ Cool       ☐ Overcast     ☐ Snowy
☐ Cold       ☐ Foggy        ☐ Windy

## Drugs / Medications

| Qty | | Description | Strength |
|---|---|---|---|
| AM | PM | | |
| | | | |
| | | | |
| | | | |
| | | | |
| | | | |
| | | | |

## Vitamins / Herbs

| Qty | | Description | Strength |
|---|---|---|---|
| AM | PM | | |
| | | | |
| | | | |
| | | | |
| | | | |
| | | | |
| | | | |

MemoryMinder©

## Physical Activity

| Activity | Hours | Mins. |
|---|---|---|
| | | |
| | | |
| | | |

## Pain / Discomfort / Skin Changes

### Scale

1 Mild
2 Moderate
3 Severe
4 Very Severe
5 Worst Possible

Mark the area where the pain occurs with the number which corresponds to the intensity of the pain.

### In general, today I felt:

☐ Good
☐ Fair
☐ Poor

## Today's Conditions and Symptoms

Check the areas which apply and explain your conditions or symptoms in the space provided. See the *Symptoms Glossary* to help you describe your conditions.

☐ *Ears / Eyes / Nose*

_____

☐ *Mouth / Throat*

_____

☐ *Head / Neck / Back*

_____

☐ *Shoulders / Arms / Hands*

_____

☐ *Chest / Heart*

_____

☐ *Respiratory System*

_____

☐ *Digestive System*

_____

☐ *Hips / Legs / Feet*

_____

☐ *Male / Female Organs*

_____

☐ *Skin*

_____

☐ *Mood*

_____

☐ *Other*

_____

_____

## Comments

_____
_____
_____
_____
_____

## Today's Diet

In columns A&B, list the nutritional facts you wish to monitor (i.e. fat, calories, sodium, sugar, protein, etc.)

| ☐ **Breakfast** | A | B |
|---|---|---|
| | | |
| | | |
| | | |
| | | |
| | | |
| Breakfast Totals | | |

| ☐ **Lunch** | | |
|---|---|---|
| | | |
| | | |
| | | |
| | | |
| | | |
| Lunch Totals | | |

| ☐ **Dinner** | | |
|---|---|---|
| | | |
| | | |
| | | |
| | | |
| | | |
| Dinner Totals | | |

| ☐ **Snacks** | | |
|---|---|---|
| | | |
| | | |
| | | |
| Snack Totals | | |

GRAND TOTALS FOR TODAY:

| A | B |
|---|---|
| | |

MemoryMinder©

| | | Date | | Day | |
| --- | --- | --- | --- | --- | --- |

|  | AM | PM |
| --- | --- | --- |
| Weight | | |
| Temperature | | |
| Blood Pressure | | |
| Sugar Level | | |
| Hours slept last night | Number of hours: | Sound ☐ Restless ☐ |
| Naps taken today | How many? | Total hours: |

## Today's Weather

- ☐ Hot
- ☐ Warm
- ☐ Cool
- ☐ Cold
- ☐ Sunny
- ☐ Cloudy
- ☐ Overcast
- ☐ Foggy
- ☐ Damp
- ☐ Rainy
- ☐ Snowy
- ☐ Windy

## Drugs / Medications

| Qty | | Description | Strength |
| --- | --- | --- | --- |
| AM | PM | | |
| | | | |
| | | | |
| | | | |
| | | | |
| | | | |
| | | | |

## Vitamins / Herbs

| Qty | | Description | Strength |
| --- | --- | --- | --- |
| AM | PM | | |
| | | | |
| | | | |
| | | | |
| | | | |
| | | | |
| | | | |

MemoryMinder©

## Physical Activity

| Activity | Hours | Mins. |
| --- | --- | --- |
| | | |
| | | |
| | | |

## Pain / Discomfort / Skin Changes

### Scale

1 Mild
2 Moderate
3 Severe
4 Very Severe
5 Worst Possible

Mark the area where the pain occurs with the number which corresponds to the intensity of the pain.

### In general, today I felt:

- ☐ Good
- ☐ Fair
- ☐ Poor

## oday's Conditions and Symptoms

eck the areas which apply and explain your conditions
symptoms in the space provided. See the *Symptoms
ossary* to help you describe your conditions.

☐ *Ears / Eyes / Nose*
_____

☐ *Mouth / Throat*
_____

☐ *Head / Neck / Back*
_____

☐ *Shoulders / Arms / Hands*
_____

☐ *Chest / Heart*
_____

☐ *Respiratory System*
_____

☐ *Digestive System*
_____

☐ *Hips / Legs / Feet*
_____

☐ *Male / Female Organs*
_____

☐ *Skin*
_____

☐ *Mood*
_____

☐ *Other*
_____

### omments
_____
_____
_____
_____

MemoryMinder©

### Today's Diet

In columns A&B, list the nutritional
facts you wish to monitor (i.e. fat,
calories, sodium, sugar, protein, etc.)

☐ **Breakfast**          A    B

Breakfast Totals

☐ **Lunch**

Lunch Totals

☐ **Dinner**

Dinner Totals

☐ **Snacks**

Snack Totals

GRAND TOTALS FOR TODAY:

| A | B |
|---|---|
|   |   |

| _____ | _____ |
| --- | --- |
| Date | Day |

|  | AM | PM |
| --- | --- | --- |
| Weight | | |
| Temperature | | |
| Blood Pressure | | |
| Sugar Level | | |
| Hours slept last night | Number of hours: | Sound ☐ Restless ☐ |
| Naps taken today | How many? | Total hours: |

## Today's Weather

- ☐ Hot
- ☐ Warm
- ☐ Cool
- ☐ Cold
- ☐ Sunny
- ☐ Cloudy
- ☐ Overcast
- ☐ Foggy
- ☐ Damp
- ☐ Rainy
- ☐ Snowy
- ☐ Windy

## Drugs / Medications

| Qty | | Description | Strength |
| --- | --- | --- | --- |
| AM | PM | | |
| | | | |
| | | | |
| | | | |
| | | | |
| | | | |
| | | | |
| | | | |

## Vitamins / Herbs

| Qty | | Description | Streng |
| --- | --- | --- | --- |
| AM | PM | | |
| | | | |
| | | | |
| | | | |
| | | | |
| | | | |
| | | | |
| | | | |

MemoryMinder©

## Physical Activity

| Activity | Hours | Mins |
| --- | --- | --- |
| | | |
| | | |
| | | |

## Pain / Discomfort / Skin Changes

### Scale

1 Mild
2 Moderate
3 Severe
4 Very Severe
5 Worst Possible

Mark the area where the pain occurs with the number which corresponds to the intensity of the pain

### In general, today I felt:

- ☐ Good
- ☐ Fair
- ☐ Poor

## Today's Conditions and Symptoms

Check the areas which apply and explain your conditions or symptoms in the space provided. See the *Symptoms Glossary* to help you describe your conditions.

☐ *Ears / Eyes / Nose*
_____
_____

☐ *Mouth / Throat*
_____
_____

☐ *Head / Neck / Back*
_____
_____

☐ *Shoulders / Arms / Hands*
_____
_____

☐ *Chest / Heart*
_____
_____

☐ *Respiratory System*
_____
_____

☐ *Digestive System*
_____
_____

☐ *Hips / Legs / Feet*
_____
_____

☐ *Male / Female Organs*
_____
_____

☐ *Skin*
_____
_____

☐ *Mood*
_____
_____

☐ *Other*
_____
_____
_____

## Comments
_____
_____
_____
_____

MemoryMinder©

## Today's Diet

In columns A&B, list the nutritional facts you wish to monitor (i.e. fat, calories, sodium, sugar, protein, etc.)

| ☐ *Breakfast* | A | B |
|---|---|---|
| | | |
| | | |
| | | |
| | | |
| | | |
| Breakfast Totals | | |

| ☐ *Lunch* | | |
|---|---|---|
| | | |
| | | |
| | | |
| | | |
| | | |
| Lunch Totals | | |

| ☐ *Dinner* | | |
|---|---|---|
| | | |
| | | |
| | | |
| | | |
| | | |
| Dinner Totals | | |

| ☐ *Snacks* | | |
|---|---|---|
| | | |
| | | |
| | | |
| Snack Totals | | |

GRAND TOTALS FOR TODAY:

| A | B |
|---|---|
| | |

| | AM | PM |
|---|---|---|
| Weight | | |
| Temperature | | |
| Blood Pressure | | |
| Sugar Level | | |
| Hours slept last night | Number of hours: | Sound ☐ Restless ☐ |
| Naps taken today | How many? | Total hours: |

_____  _____
Date                              Day

## *Today's Weather*

☐ Hot     ☐ Sunny      ☐ Damp
☐ Warm    ☐ Cloudy     ☐ Rainy
☐ Cool    ☐ Overcast   ☐ Snowy
☐ Cold    ☐ Foggy      ☐ Windy

## *Drugs / Medications*

| Qty | | Description | Strength |
|---|---|---|---|
| AM | PM | | |
| | | | |
| | | | |
| | | | |
| | | | |
| | | | |
| | | | |
| | | | |

## *Vitamins / Herbs*

| Qty | | Description | Strength |
|---|---|---|---|
| AM | PM | | |
| | | | |
| | | | |
| | | | |
| | | | |
| | | | |
| | | | |

MemoryMinder©

## *Physical Activity*

| Activity | Hours | Mins. |
|---|---|---|
| | | |
| | | |
| | | |

## *Pain / Discomfort / Skin Changes*

### Scale

1 Mild
2 Moderate
3 Severe
4 Very Severe
5 Worst Possible

Mark the area where the pain occurs with the number which corresponds to the intensity of the pain.

## *In general, today I felt:*

☐ Good
☐ Fair
☐ Poor

# oday's Conditions and Symptoms

eck the areas which apply and explain your conditions
 symptoms in the space provided. See the *Symptoms*
*ossary* to help you describe your conditions.

☐ *Ears / Eyes / Nose*

_____

☐ *Mouth / Throat*

_____

☐ *Head / Neck / Back*

_____

☐ *Shoulders / Arms / Hands*

_____

☐ *Chest / Heart*

_____

☐ *Respiratory System*

_____

☐ *Digestive System*

_____

☐ *Hips / Legs / Feet*

_____

☐ *Male / Female Organs*

_____

☐ *Skin*

_____

☐ *Mood*

_____

☐ *Other*

_____
_____

## omments
_____
_____
_____
_____

---

## Today's Diet

In columns A&B, list the nutritional
facts you wish to monitor (i.e. fat,
calories, sodium, sugar, protein, etc.)

☐ **Breakfast**

| | A | B |
|---|---|---|
| | | |
| | | |
| | | |
| | | |
| | | |
| Breakfast Totals | | |

☐ **Lunch**

| | | |
|---|---|---|
| | | |
| | | |
| | | |
| | | |
| Lunch Totals | | |

☐ **Dinner**

| | | |
|---|---|---|
| | | |
| | | |
| | | |
| | | |
| | | |
| Dinner Totals | | |

☐ **Snacks**

| | | |
|---|---|---|
| | | |
| | | |
| Snack Totals | | |

GRAND TOTALS FOR TODAY:

| A | B |
|---|---|
| | |

MemoryMinder©

| | | AM | PM |
|---|---|---|---|
| _____ _____ | Weight | | |
| Date Day | Temperature | | |
| | Blood Pressure | | |
| | Sugar Level | | |
| | Hours slept last night | Number of hours: | Sound ☐ Restless ☐ |
| | Naps taken today | How many? | Total hours: |

## Today's Weather

☐ Hot    ☐ Sunny    ☐ Damp
☐ Warm    ☐ Cloudy    ☐ Rainy
☐ Cool    ☐ Overcast    ☐ Snowy
☐ Cold    ☐ Foggy    ☐ Windy

## Drugs / Medications

| Qty | | Description | Strength |
|---|---|---|---|
| AM | PM | | |
| | | | |
| | | | |
| | | | |
| | | | |
| | | | |
| | | | |

## Vitamins / Herbs

| Qty | | Description | Strengt |
|---|---|---|---|
| AM | PM | | |
| | | | |
| | | | |
| | | | |
| | | | |
| | | | |
| | | | |

MemoryMinder©

## Physical Activity

| Activity | Hours | Mins |
|---|---|---|
| | | |
| | | |
| | | |

## Pain / Discomfort / Skin Changes

### Scale

1 Mild
2 Moderate
3 Severe
4 Very Severe
5 Worst Possible

Mark the area where the pain occurs with the number which corresponds to the intensity of the pain.

### In general, today I felt:

☐ Good

☐ Fair

☐ Poor

## Today's Conditions and Symptoms

Check the areas which apply and explain your conditions
or symptoms in the space provided. See the *Symptoms
Glossary* to help you describe your conditions.

☐ *Ears / Eyes / Nose*

_____

☐ *Mouth / Throat*

_____

☐ *Head / Neck / Back*

_____

☐ *Shoulders / Arms / Hands*

_____

☐ *Chest / Heart*

_____

☐ *Respiratory System*

_____

☐ *Digestive System*

_____

☐ *Hips / Legs / Feet*

_____

☐ *Male / Female Organs*

_____

☐ *Skin*

_____

☐ *Mood*

_____

☐ *Other*

_____
_____

## Comments

_____
_____
_____
_____

## Today's Diet

In columns A&B, list the nutritional
facts you wish to monitor (i.e. fat,
calories, sodium, sugar, protein, etc.)

| ☐ **Breakfast** | A | B |
|---|---|---|
| | | |
| | | |
| | | |
| | | |
| Breakfast Totals | | |

| ☐ **Lunch** | | |
|---|---|---|
| | | |
| | | |
| | | |
| | | |
| Lunch Totals | | |

| ☐ **Dinner** | | |
|---|---|---|
| | | |
| | | |
| | | |
| | | |
| Dinner Totals | | |

| ☐ **Snacks** | | |
|---|---|---|
| | | |
| | | |
| Snack Totals | | |

GRAND TOTALS FOR TODAY:

| A | B |
|---|---|
| | |

MemoryMinder©

| | Date | Day |
|---|---|---|

## Today's Weather

- ☐ Hot
- ☐ Warm
- ☐ Cool
- ☐ Cold
- ☐ Sunny
- ☐ Cloudy
- ☐ Overcast
- ☐ Foggy
- ☐ Damp
- ☐ Rainy
- ☐ Snowy
- ☐ Windy

| | AM | PM |
|---|---|---|
| Weight | | |
| Temperature | | |
| Blood Pressure | | |
| Sugar Level | | |
| Hours slept last night | Number of hours: | Sound ☐ Restless ☐ |
| Naps taken today | How many? | Total hours: |

## Drugs / Medications

| Qty | | Description | Strength |
|---|---|---|---|
| AM | PM | | |
| | | | |
| | | | |
| | | | |
| | | | |
| | | | |
| | | | |

## Vitamins / Herbs

| Qty | | Description | Strength |
|---|---|---|---|
| AM | PM | | |
| | | | |
| | | | |
| | | | |
| | | | |
| | | | |
| | | | |

MemoryMinder©

## Physical Activity

| Activity | Hours | Mins. |
|---|---|---|
| | | |
| | | |
| | | |

## Pain / Discomfort / Skin Changes

### Scale

1 Mild
2 Moderate
3 Severe
4 Very Severe
5 Worst Possible

Mark the area where the pain occurs with the number which corresponds to the intensity of the pain.

### In general, today I felt:

- ☐ Good
- ☐ Fair
- ☐ Poor

# Today's Conditions and Symptoms

Check the areas which apply and explain your conditions or symptoms in the space provided. See the *Symptoms Glossary* to help you describe your conditions.

☐ **Ears / Eyes / Nose**
_____

☐ **Mouth / Throat**
_____

☐ **Head / Neck / Back**
_____

☐ **Shoulders / Arms / Hands**
_____

☐ **Chest / Heart**
_____

☐ **Respiratory System**
_____

☐ **Digestive System**
_____

☐ **Hips / Legs / Feet**
_____

☐ **Male / Female Organs**
_____

☐ **Skin**
_____

☐ **Mood**
_____

☐ **Other**
_____
_____

## Comments
_____
_____
_____
_____

# Today's Diet

In columns A&B, list the nutritional facts you wish to monitor (i.e. fat, calories, sodium, sugar, protein, etc.)

| ☐ **Breakfast** | A | B |
|---|---|---|
| | | |
| | | |
| | | |
| | | |
| | | |
| Breakfast Totals | | |

| ☐ **Lunch** | | |
|---|---|---|
| | | |
| | | |
| | | |
| | | |
| | | |
| Lunch Totals | | |

| ☐ **Dinner** | | |
|---|---|---|
| | | |
| | | |
| | | |
| | | |
| | | |
| Dinner Totals | | |

| ☐ **Snacks** | | |
|---|---|---|
| | | |
| | | |
| | | |
| Snack Totals | | |

GRAND TOTALS FOR TODAY:

| A | B |
|---|---|
| | |

MemoryMinder©

| | | AM | PM |
|---|---|---|---|
| Date _____ Day _____ | | | |

| | | AM | PM |
|---|---|---|---|
| Weight | | | |
| Temperature | | | |
| Blood Pressure | | / | / |
| Sugar Level | | | |
| Hours slept last night | Number of hours: | | Sound ☐ Restless ☐ |
| Naps taken today | How many? | | Total hours: |

## Today's Weather

☐ Hot  ☐ Sunny  ☐ Damp
☐ Warm  ☐ Cloudy  ☐ Rainy
☐ Cool  ☐ Overcast  ☐ Snowy
☐ Cold  ☐ Foggy  ☐ Windy

## Drugs / Medications

| Qty | | Description | Strength |
|---|---|---|---|
| AM | PM | | |
| | | | |
| | | | |
| | | | |
| | | | |
| | | | |
| | | | |

## Vitamins / Herbs

| Qty | | Description | Strength |
|---|---|---|---|
| AM | PM | | |
| | | | |
| | | | |
| | | | |
| | | | |
| | | | |
| | | | |

MemoryMinder©

## Physical Activity

| Activity | Hours | Mins. |
|---|---|---|
| | | |
| | | |
| | | |

## Pain / Discomfort / Skin Changes

### Scale

1 Mild
2 Moderate
3 Severe
4 Very Severe
5 Worst Possible

Mark the area where the pain occurs with the number which corresponds to the intensity of the pain.

### In general, today I felt:

☐ Good
☐ Fair
☐ Poor

# Today's Conditions and Symptoms

Check the areas which apply and explain your conditions symptoms in the space provided. See the *Symptoms Glossary* to help you describe your conditions.

☐ *Ears / Eyes / Nose*
_____

☐ *Mouth / Throat*
_____

☐ *Head / Neck / Back*
_____

☐ *Shoulders / Arms / Hands*
_____

☐ *Chest / Heart*
_____

☐ *Respiratory System*
_____

☐ *Digestive System*
_____

☐ *Hips / Legs / Feet*
_____

☐ *Male / Female Organs*
_____

☐ *Skin*
_____

☐ *Mood*
_____

☐ *Other*
_____
_____

## Comments
_____
_____
_____
_____

---

## Today's Diet

In columns A&B, list the nutritional facts you wish to monitor (i.e. fat, calories, sodium, sugar, protein, etc.)

☐ **Breakfast**      A    B

Breakfast Totals

☐ **Lunch**

Lunch Totals

☐ **Dinner**

Dinner Totals

☐ **Snacks**

Snack Totals

GRAND TOTALS FOR TODAY:

| A | B |
|---|---|
|   |   |

MemoryMinder©

| | AM | PM |
|---|---|---|
| Weight | | |
| Temperature | | |
| Blood Pressure | | |
| Sugar Level | | |

_____  _____
Date                        Day

## Today's Weather

- ☐ Hot
- ☐ Warm
- ☐ Cool
- ☐ Cold
- ☐ Sunny
- ☐ Cloudy
- ☐ Overcast
- ☐ Foggy
- ☐ Damp
- ☐ Rainy
- ☐ Snowy
- ☐ Windy

Hours slept last night — Number of hours: — Sound ☐ Restless ☐

Naps taken today — How many: — Total hours:

## Drugs / Medications

| Qty AM | PM | Description | Strength |
|---|---|---|---|
| | | | |
| | | | |
| | | | |
| | | | |
| | | | |
| | | | |

## Vitamins / Herbs

| Qty AM | PM | Description | Strengt |
|---|---|---|---|
| | | | |
| | | | |
| | | | |
| | | | |
| | | | |
| | | | |

MemoryMinder©

## Physical Activity

| Activity | Hours | Mins. |
|---|---|---|
| | | |
| | | |
| | | |

## Pain / Discomfort / Skin Changes

### Scale

1 Mild
2 Moderate
3 Severe
4 Very Severe
5 Worst Possible

Mark the area where the pain occurs with the number which corresponds to the intensity of the pain.

## In general, today I felt:

- ☐ Good
- ☐ Fair
- ☐ Poor

## Today's Conditions and Symptoms

Check the areas which apply and explain your conditions or symptoms in the space provided. See the *Symptoms Glossary* to help you describe your conditions.

☐ *Ears / Eyes / Nose*

_____

☐ *Mouth / Throat*

_____

☐ *Head / Neck / Back*

_____

☐ *Shoulders / Arms / Hands*

_____

☐ *Chest / Heart*

_____

☐ *Respiratory System*

_____

☐ *Digestive System*

_____

☐ *Hips / Legs / Feet*

_____

☐ *Male / Female Organs*

_____

☐ *Skin*

_____

☐ *Mood*

_____

☐ *Other*

_____

_____

## Comments

_____

_____

_____

_____

_____

MemoryMinder©

## Today's Diet

In columns A&B, list the nutritional facts you wish to monitor (i.e. fat, calories, sodium, sugar, protein, etc.)

☐ *Breakfast*

| | A | B |
|---|---|---|
| | | |
| | | |
| | | |
| | | |
| Breakfast Totals | | |

☐ *Lunch*

| | A | B |
|---|---|---|
| | | |
| | | |
| | | |
| | | |
| Lunch Totals | | |

☐ *Dinner*

| | A | B |
|---|---|---|
| | | |
| | | |
| | | |
| | | |
| Dinner Totals | | |

☐ *Snacks*

| | A | B |
|---|---|---|
| | | |
| | | |
| Snack Totals | | |

GRAND TOTALS FOR TODAY:

| A | B |
|---|---|
| | |

| | | AM | PM |
|---|---|---|---|
| | Date _____ _____ Day | | |

## Today's Weather

| | | |
|---|---|---|
| ☐ Hot | ☐ Sunny | ☐ Damp |
| ☐ Warm | ☐ Cloudy | ☐ Rainy |
| ☐ Cool | ☐ Overcast | ☐ Snowy |
| ☐ Cold | ☐ Foggy | ☐ Windy |

| | AM | PM |
|---|---|---|
| Weight | | |
| Temperature | | |
| Blood Pressure | | |
| Sugar Level | | |
| Hours slept last night | Number of hours: | Sound ☐ Restless ☐ |
| Naps taken today | How many? | Total hours: |

## Drugs / Medications

| Qty | | Description | Strength |
|---|---|---|---|
| AM | PM | | |
| | | | |
| | | | |
| | | | |
| | | | |
| | | | |
| | | | |

## Vitamins / Herbs

| Qty | | Description | Strength |
|---|---|---|---|
| AM | PM | | |
| | | | |
| | | | |
| | | | |
| | | | |
| | | | |
| | | | |

MemoryMinder©

## Physical Activity

| Activity | Hours | Mins. |
|---|---|---|
| | | |
| | | |
| | | |

## Pain / Discomfort / Skin Changes

### Scale

1 Mild
2 Moderate
3 Severe
4 Very Severe
5 Worst Possible

Mark the area where the pain occurs with the number which corresponds to the intensity of the pain.

### In general, today I felt:

☐ Good

☐ Fair

☐ Poor

## Today's Conditions and Symptoms

Check the areas which apply and explain your conditions or symptoms in the space provided. See the *Symptoms Glossary* to help you describe your conditions.

☐ *Ears / Eyes / Nose*

_____

☐ *Mouth / Throat*

_____

☐ *Head / Neck / Back*

_____

☐ *Shoulders / Arms / Hands*

_____

☐ *Chest / Heart*

_____

☐ *Respiratory System*

_____

☐ *Digestive System*

_____

☐ *Hips / Legs / Feet*

_____

☐ *Male / Female Organs*

_____

☐ *Skin*

_____

☐ *Mood*

_____

☐ *Other*

_____

_____

## Comments

_____
_____
_____
_____

MemoryMinder©

## Today's Diet

In columns A&B, list the nutritional facts you wish to monitor (i.e. fat, calories, sodium, sugar, protein, etc.)

☐ *Breakfast*    A    B

Breakfast Totals

☐ *Lunch*

Lunch Totals

☐ *Dinner*

Dinner Totals

☐ *Snacks*

Snack Totals

GRAND TOTALS FOR TODAY:

| A | B |
|---|---|
|   |   |

| | AM | PM |
|---|---|---|
| Weight | | |
| Temperature | | |
| Blood Pressure | | |
| Sugar Level | | |
| Hours slept last night | Number of hours: | Sound ☐ Restless ☐ |
| Naps taken today | How many? | Total hours: |

_____  _____
Date             Day

## Today's Weather

☐ Hot      ☐ Sunny     ☐ Damp
☐ Warm     ☐ Cloudy    ☐ Rainy
☐ Cool     ☐ Overcast  ☐ Snowy
☐ Cold     ☐ Foggy     ☐ Windy

## Drugs / Medications

| Qty | | Description | Strength |
|---|---|---|---|
| AM | PM | | |
| | | | |
| | | | |
| | | | |
| | | | |
| | | | |
| | | | |

## Vitamins / Herbs

| Qty | | Description | Strength |
|---|---|---|---|
| AM | PM | | |
| | | | |
| | | | |
| | | | |
| | | | |
| | | | |
| | | | |

MemoryMinder©

## Physical Activity

| Activity | Hours | Mins. |
|---|---|---|
| | | |
| | | |
| | | |
| | | |

## Pain / Discomfort / Skin Changes

### Scale

1 Mild
2 Moderate
3 Severe
4 Very Severe
5 Worst Possible

Mark the area where the pain occurs with the number which corresponds to the intensity of the pain.

### In general, today I felt:

☐ Good
☐ Fair
☐ Poor

## Today's Conditions and Symptoms

Check the areas which apply and explain your conditions & symptoms in the space provided. See the *Symptoms Glossary* to help you describe your conditions.

☐ *Ears / Eyes / Nose*

_____

☐ *Mouth / Throat*

_____

☐ *Head / Neck / Back*

_____

☐ *Shoulders / Arms / Hands*

_____

☐ *Chest / Heart*

_____

☐ *Respiratory System*

_____

☐ *Digestive System*

_____

☐ *Hips / Legs / Feet*

_____

☐ *Male / Female Organs*

_____

☐ *Skin*

_____

☐ *Mood*

_____

☐ *Other*

_____
_____

## Comments

_____
_____
_____
_____
_____

MemoryMinder©

## Today's Diet

In columns A&B, list the nutritional facts you wish to monitor (i.e. fat, calories, sodium, sugar, protein, etc.)

☐ **Breakfast**

| | A | B |
|---|---|---|
| | | |
| | | |
| | | |
| | | |
| | | |
| Breakfast Totals | | |

☐ **Lunch**

| | A | B |
|---|---|---|
| | | |
| | | |
| | | |
| | | |
| | | |
| Lunch Totals | | |

☐ **Dinner**

| | A | B |
|---|---|---|
| | | |
| | | |
| | | |
| | | |
| | | |
| Dinner Totals | | |

☐ **Snacks**

| | A | B |
|---|---|---|
| | | |
| | | |
| | | |
| Snack Totals | | |

GRAND TOTALS FOR TODAY:

| A | B |
|---|---|
| | |

_____ _____
Date          Day

| | AM | PM |
|---|---|---|
| Weight | | |
| Temperature | | |
| Blood Pressure | | |
| Sugar Level | | |
| Hours slept last night | Number of hours: | Sound ☐ Restless ☐ |
| Naps taken today | How many? | Total hours: |

## Today's Weather

☐ Hot      ☐ Sunny      ☐ Damp
☐ Warm     ☐ Cloudy     ☐ Rainy
☐ Cool     ☐ Overcast   ☐ Snowy
☐ Cold     ☐ Foggy      ☐ Windy

## Drugs / Medications

| Qty | | Description | Strength |
|---|---|---|---|
| AM | PM | | |
| | | | |
| | | | |
| | | | |
| | | | |
| | | | |
| | | | |
| | | | |

## Vitamins / Herbs

| Qty | | Description | Streng |
|---|---|---|---|
| AM | PM | | |
| | | | |
| | | | |
| | | | |
| | | | |
| | | | |

MemoryMinder©

## Physical Activity

| Activity | Hours | Mins |
|---|---|---|
| | | |
| | | |
| | | |

## Pain / Discomfort / Skin Changes

### Scale

1 Mild
2 Moderate
3 Severe
4 Very Severe
5 Worst Possible

Mark the area where the pain occurs with the number which corresponds to the intensity of the pain

## In general, today I felt:

☐ Good

☐ Fair

☐ Poor

## Today's Conditions and Symptoms

Check the areas which apply and explain your conditions or symptoms in the space provided. See the *Symptoms Glossary* to help you describe your conditions.

☐ *Ears / Eyes / Nose*
_____

☐ *Mouth / Throat*
_____

☐ *Head / Neck / Back*
_____

☐ *Shoulders / Arms / Hands*
_____

☐ *Chest / Heart*
_____

☐ *Respiratory System*
_____

☐ *Digestive System*
_____

☐ *Hips / Legs / Feet*
_____

☐ *Male / Female Organs*
_____

☐ *Skin*
_____

☐ *Mood*
_____

☐ *Other*
_____

## Comments
_____
_____
_____
_____

## Today's Diet

In columns A&B, list the nutritional facts you wish to monitor (i.e. fat, calories, sodium, sugar, protein, etc.)

| ☐ **Breakfast** | A | B |
|---|---|---|
| | | |
| | | |
| | | |
| | | |
| | | |
| Breakfast Totals | | |

| ☐ **Lunch** | | |
|---|---|---|
| | | |
| | | |
| | | |
| | | |
| | | |
| Lunch Totals | | |

| ☐ **Dinner** | | |
|---|---|---|
| | | |
| | | |
| | | |
| | | |
| | | |
| Dinner Totals | | |

| ☐ **Snacks** | | |
|---|---|---|
| | | |
| | | |
| | | |
| Snack Totals | | |

GRAND TOTALS FOR TODAY:

| A | B |
|---|---|
| | |

MemoryMinder©

| | AM | PM |
|---|---|---|
| Weight | | |
| Temperature | | |
| Blood Pressure | | |
| Sugar Level | | |
| Hours slept last night | Number of hours: | Sound ☐ Restless ☐ |
| Naps taken today | How many? | Total hours: |

_____ _____
Date          Day

## Today's Weather

☐ Hot     ☐ Sunny     ☐ Damp
☐ Warm    ☐ Cloudy    ☐ Rainy
☐ Cool    ☐ Overcast  ☐ Snowy
☐ Cold    ☐ Foggy     ☐ Windy

## Drugs / Medications

| Qty | | Description | Strength |
|---|---|---|---|
| AM | PM | | |
| | | | |
| | | | |
| | | | |
| | | | |
| | | | |
| | | | |

## Vitamins / Herbs

| Qty | | Description | Strength |
|---|---|---|---|
| AM | PM | | |
| | | | |
| | | | |
| | | | |
| | | | |
| | | | |
| | | | |

MemoryMinder©

## Physical Activity

| Activity | Hours | Mins. |
|---|---|---|
| | | |
| | | |
| | | |
| | | |

## Pain / Discomfort / Skin Changes

### Scale

1 Mild
2 Moderate
3 Severe
4 Very Severe
5 Worst Possible

Mark the area where the pain occurs with the number which corresponds to the intensity of the pain.

### In general, today I felt:

☐ Good
☐ Fair
☐ Poor

## Today's Conditions and Symptoms

Check the areas which apply and explain your conditions & symptoms in the space provided. See the *Symptoms Glossary* to help you describe your conditions.

☐ *Ears / Eyes / Nose*
_____

☐ *Mouth / Throat*
_____

☐ *Head / Neck / Back*
_____

☐ *Shoulders / Arms / Hands*
_____

☐ *Chest / Heart*
_____

☐ *Respiratory System*
_____

☐ *Digestive System*
_____

☐ *Hips / Legs / Feet*
_____

☐ *Male / Female Organs*
_____

☐ *Skin*
_____

☐ *Mood*
_____

☐ *Other*
_____

## Comments
_____
_____
_____
_____

## Today's Diet

In columns A&B, list the nutritional facts you wish to monitor (i.e. fat, calories, sodium, sugar, protein, etc.)

| ☐ **Breakfast** | A | B |
|---|---|---|
| | | |
| | | |
| | | |
| | | |
| | | |
| Breakfast Totals | | |

| ☐ **Lunch** | | |
|---|---|---|
| | | |
| | | |
| | | |
| | | |
| | | |
| Lunch Totals | | |

| ☐ **Dinner** | | |
|---|---|---|
| | | |
| | | |
| | | |
| | | |
| | | |
| Dinner Totals | | |

| ☐ **Snacks** | | |
|---|---|---|
| | | |
| | | |
| | | |
| Snack Totals | | |

GRAND TOTALS FOR TODAY:

| A | B |
|---|---|
| | |

MemoryMinder©

| | | AM | PM |
|---|---|---|---|
| Weight | | | |
| Temperature | | | |
| Blood Pressure | | / | / |
| Sugar Level | | | |
| Hours slept last night | | Number of hours: | Sound ☐ Restless ☐ |
| Naps taken today | | How many? | Total hours: |

_____  _____
Date                Day

## Today's Weather

☐ Hot    ☐ Sunny    ☐ Damp
☐ Warm    ☐ Cloudy    ☐ Rainy
☐ Cool    ☐ Overcast    ☐ Snowy
☐ Cold    ☐ Foggy    ☐ Windy

## Drugs / Medications

| Qty | | Description | Strength |
|---|---|---|---|
| AM | PM | | |
| | | | |
| | | | |
| | | | |
| | | | |
| | | | |
| | | | |
| | | | |

## Vitamins / Herbs

| Qty | | Description | Strengt |
|---|---|---|---|
| AM | PM | | |
| | | | |
| | | | |
| | | | |
| | | | |
| | | | |
| | | | |
| | | | |

MemoryMinder©

## Physical Activity

| Activity | Hours | Mins. |
|---|---|---|
| | | |
| | | |
| | | |

## Pain / Discomfort / Skin Changes

### Scale

1 Mild
2 Moderate
3 Severe
4 Very Severe
5 Worst Possible

Mark the area where the pain occurs with the number which corresponds to the intensity of the pain.

### In general, today I felt:

☐ Good
☐ Fair
☐ Poor

## Today's Conditions and Symptoms

Check the areas which apply and explain your conditions or symptoms in the space provided. See the *Symptoms Glossary* to help you describe your conditions.

☐ *Ears / Eyes / Nose*

_____

☐ *Mouth / Throat*

_____

☐ *Head / Neck / Back*

_____

☐ *Shoulders / Arms / Hands*

_____

☐ *Chest / Heart*

_____

☐ *Respiratory System*

_____

☐ *Digestive System*

_____

☐ *Hips / Legs / Feet*

_____

☐ *Male / Female Organs*

_____

☐ *Skin*

_____

☐ *Mood*

_____

☐ *Other*

_____
_____

## Comments

_____
_____
_____
_____

## Today's Diet

In columns A&B, list the nutritional facts you wish to monitor (i.e. fat, calories, sodium, sugar, protein, etc.)

| ☐ **Breakfast** | A | B |
|---|---|---|
| | | |
| | | |
| | | |
| | | |
| Breakfast Totals | | |

| ☐ **Lunch** | | |
|---|---|---|
| | | |
| | | |
| | | |
| | | |
| | | |
| Lunch Totals | | |

| ☐ **Dinner** | | |
|---|---|---|
| | | |
| | | |
| | | |
| | | |
| | | |
| | | |
| Dinner Totals | | |

| ☐ **Snacks** | | |
|---|---|---|
| | | |
| | | |
| | | |
| Snack Totals | | |

| GRAND TOTALS FOR TODAY: | |
|---|---|
| A | B |

MemoryMinder©

| | Date | | Day | | AM | PM |
|---|---|---|---|---|---|---|

| | AM | PM |
|---|---|---|
| Weight | | |
| Temperature | | |
| Blood Pressure | | |
| Sugar Level | | |
| Hours slept last night | Number of hours: | Sound ☐ Restless ☐ |
| Naps taken today | How many? | Total hours: |

## Today's Weather

☐ Hot  ☐ Sunny  ☐ Damp
☐ Warm  ☐ Cloudy  ☐ Rainy
☐ Cool  ☐ Overcast  ☐ Snowy
☐ Cold  ☐ Foggy  ☐ Windy

## Drugs / Medications

| Qty | | Description | Strength |
|---|---|---|---|
| AM | PM | | |
| | | | |
| | | | |
| | | | |
| | | | |
| | | | |
| | | | |

## Vitamins / Herbs

| Qty | | Description | Strength |
|---|---|---|---|
| AM | PM | | |
| | | | |
| | | | |
| | | | |
| | | | |
| | | | |

MemoryMinder©

## Physical Activity

| Activity | Hours | Mins. |
|---|---|---|
| | | |
| | | |
| | | |

## Pain / Discomfort / Skin Changes

### Scale

1 Mild
2 Moderate
3 Severe
4 Very Severe
5 Worst Possible

Mark the area where the pain occurs with the number which corresponds to the intensity of the pain.

### In general, today I felt:

☐ Good
☐ Fair
☐ Poor

# Today's Conditions and Symptoms

Check the areas which apply and explain your conditions or symptoms in the space provided. See the *Symptoms Glossary* to help you describe your conditions.

☐ *Ears / Eyes / Nose*
_____

☐ *Mouth / Throat*
_____

☐ *Head / Neck / Back*
_____

☐ *Shoulders / Arms / Hands*
_____

☐ *Chest / Heart*
_____

☐ *Respiratory System*
_____

☐ *Digestive System*
_____

☐ *Hips / Legs / Feet*
_____

☐ *Male / Female Organs*
_____

☐ *Skin*
_____

☐ *Mood*
_____

☐ *Other*
_____
_____

# Comments
_____
_____
_____
_____

MemoryMinder©

# Today's Diet

In columns A&B, list the nutritional facts you wish to monitor (i.e. fat, calories, sodium, sugar, protein, etc.)

| ☐ **Breakfast** | A | B |
|---|---|---|
| | | |
| | | |
| | | |
| | | |
| | | |
| Breakfast Totals | | |

| ☐ **Lunch** | | |
|---|---|---|
| | | |
| | | |
| | | |
| | | |
| | | |
| Lunch Totals | | |

| ☐ **Dinner** | | |
|---|---|---|
| | | |
| | | |
| | | |
| | | |
| | | |
| Dinner Totals | | |

| ☐ **Snacks** | | |
|---|---|---|
| | | |
| | | |
| | | |
| Snack Totals | | |

GRAND TOTALS FOR TODAY:

| A | B |
|---|---|
| | |

_____   _____
Date                Day

| | AM | PM |
|---|---|---|
| Weight | | |
| Temperature | | |
| Blood Pressure | | |
| Sugar Level | | |

## Today's Weather

- [ ] Hot
- [ ] Warm
- [ ] Cool
- [ ] Cold
- [ ] Sunny
- [ ] Cloudy
- [ ] Overcast
- [ ] Foggy
- [ ] Damp
- [ ] Rainy
- [ ] Snowy
- [ ] Windy

| Hours slept last night | Number of hours: | | Sound [ ] Restless [ ] |
| Naps taken today | How many? | | Total hours: |

## Drugs / Medications

| Qty | | Description | Strength |
|---|---|---|---|
| AM | PM | | |
| | | | |
| | | | |
| | | | |
| | | | |
| | | | |
| | | | |

## Vitamins / Herbs

| Qty | | Description | Strength |
|---|---|---|---|
| AM | PM | | |
| | | | |
| | | | |
| | | | |
| | | | |
| | | | |

MemoryMinder©

## Physical Activity

| Activity | Hours | Mins. |
|---|---|---|
| | | |
| | | |
| | | |
| | | |

## Pain / Discomfort / Skin Changes

### Scale

1 Mild
2 Moderate
3 Severe
4 Very Severe
5 Worst Possible

Mark the area where the pain occurs with the number which corresponds to the intensity of the pain.

### In general, today I felt:

- [ ] Good
- [ ] Fair
- [ ] Poor

## Today's Conditions and Symptoms

Check the areas which apply and explain your conditions or symptoms in the space provided. See the *Symptoms Glossary* to help you describe your conditions.

☐ *Ears / Eyes / Nose*
_____

☐ *Mouth / Throat*
_____

☐ *Head / Neck / Back*
_____

☐ *Shoulders / Arms / Hands*
_____

☐ *Chest / Heart*
_____

☐ *Respiratory System*
_____

☐ *Digestive System*
_____

☐ *Hips / Legs / Feet*
_____

☐ *Male / Female Organs*
_____

☐ *Skin*
_____

☐ *Mood*
_____

☐ *Other*
_____

## Comments
_____
_____
_____
_____

## Today's Diet

In columns A&B, list the nutritional facts you wish to monitor (i.e. fat, calories, sodium, sugar, protein, etc.)

| ☐ **Breakfast** | A | B |
|---|---|---|
| | | |
| | | |
| | | |
| | | |
| | | |
| Breakfast Totals | | |

| ☐ **Lunch** | | |
|---|---|---|
| | | |
| | | |
| | | |
| | | |
| | | |
| Lunch Totals | | |

| ☐ **Dinner** | | |
|---|---|---|
| | | |
| | | |
| | | |
| | | |
| | | |
| Dinner Totals | | |

| ☐ **Snacks** | | |
|---|---|---|
| | | |
| | | |
| | | |
| Snack Totals | | |

GRAND TOTALS FOR TODAY:

| A | B |
|---|---|
| | |

MemoryMinder©

| | Date | Day | | AM | PM |
|---|---|---|---|---|---|
| | | | Weight | | |
| | | | Temperature | | |
| | | | Blood Pressure | | |
| | | | Sugar Level | | |
| | | | Hours slept last night | Number of hours: | Sound ☐ Restless ☐ |
| | | | Naps taken today | How many? | Total hours: |

## Today's Weather

☐ Hot  ☐ Sunny  ☐ Damp
☐ Warm  ☐ Cloudy  ☐ Rainy
☐ Cool  ☐ Overcast  ☐ Snowy
☐ Cold  ☐ Foggy  ☐ Windy

## Drugs / Medications

| Qty | | Description | Strength |
|---|---|---|---|
| AM | PM | | |
| | | | |
| | | | |
| | | | |
| | | | |
| | | | |
| | | | |

## Vitamins / Herbs

| Qty | | Description | Strength |
|---|---|---|---|
| AM | PM | | |
| | | | |
| | | | |
| | | | |
| | | | |
| | | | |
| | | | |

MemoryMinder©

## Physical Activity

| Activity | Hours | Mins. |
|---|---|---|
| | | |
| | | |
| | | |

## Pain / Discomfort / Skin Changes

### Scale

1 Mild
2 Moderate
3 Severe
4 Very Severe
5 Worst Possible

Mark the area where the pain occurs with the number which corresponds to the intensity of the pain.

### In general, today I felt:

☐ Good
☐ Fair
☐ Poor

# Today's Conditions and Symptoms

Check the areas which apply and explain your conditions
or symptoms in the space provided. See the *Symptoms
Glossary* to help you describe your conditions.

☐ *Ears / Eyes / Nose*
_____

☐ *Mouth / Throat*
_____

☐ *Head / Neck / Back*
_____

☐ *Shoulders / Arms / Hands*
_____

☐ *Chest / Heart*
_____

☐ *Respiratory System*
_____

☐ *Digestive System*
_____

☐ *Hips / Legs / Feet*
_____

☐ *Male / Female Organs*
_____

☐ *Skin*
_____

☐ *Mood*
_____

☐ *Other*
_____
_____

## Comments
_____
_____
_____
_____

# Today's Diet

In columns A&B, list the nutritional
facts you wish to monitor (i.e. fat,
calories, sodium, sugar, protein, etc.)

☐ **Breakfast**

| | A | B |
|---|---|---|
| | | |
| | | |
| | | |
| | | |
| | | |
| Breakfast Totals | | |

☐ **Lunch**

| | A | B |
|---|---|---|
| | | |
| | | |
| | | |
| | | |
| | | |
| Lunch Totals | | |

☐ **Dinner**

| | A | B |
|---|---|---|
| | | |
| | | |
| | | |
| | | |
| | | |
| Dinner Totals | | |

☐ **Snacks**

| | A | B |
|---|---|---|
| | | |
| | | |
| | | |
| Snack Totals | | |

GRAND TOTALS FOR TODAY:

| A | B |
|---|---|
| | |

MemoryMinder©

| | | AM | PM |
|---|---|---|---|
| Weight | | | |
| Temperature | | | |
| Blood Pressure | | | |
| Sugar Level | | | |
| Hours slept last night | Number of hours: | | Sound ☐ Restless ☐ |
| Naps taken today | How many? | | Total hours: |

_____  _____
Date                    Day

## Today's Weather

☐ Hot      ☐ Sunny      ☐ Damp
☐ Warm     ☐ Cloudy     ☐ Rainy
☐ Cool     ☐ Overcast   ☐ Snowy
☐ Cold     ☐ Foggy      ☐ Windy

## Drugs / Medications

| Qty | | Description | Strength |
|---|---|---|---|
| AM | PM | | |
| | | | |
| | | | |
| | | | |
| | | | |
| | | | |
| | | | |

## Vitamins / Herbs

| Qty | | Description | Strength |
|---|---|---|---|
| AM | PM | | |
| | | | |
| | | | |
| | | | |
| | | | |
| | | | |
| | | | |

MemoryMinder©

## Physical Activity

| Activity | Hours | Mins. |
|---|---|---|
| | | |
| | | |
| | | |

## Pain / Discomfort / Skin Changes

### Scale

1 Mild
2 Moderate
3 Severe
4 Very Severe
5 Worst Possible

Mark the area where the pain occurs with the number which corresponds to the intensity of the pain.

### In general, today I felt:

☐ Good
☐ Fair
☐ Poor

# Today's Conditions and Symptoms

Check the areas which apply and explain your conditions symptoms in the space provided. See the *Symptoms Glossary* to help you describe your conditions.

☐ *Ears / Eyes / Nose*
_____

☐ *Mouth / Throat*
_____

☐ *Head / Neck / Back*
_____

☐ *Shoulders / Arms / Hands*
_____

☐ *Chest / Heart*
_____

☐ *Respiratory System*
_____

☐ *Digestive System*
_____

☐ *Hips / Legs / Feet*
_____

☐ *Male / Female Organs*
_____

☐ *Skin*
_____

☐ *Mood*
_____

☐ *Other*
_____
_____

## Comments
_____
_____
_____
_____

# Today's Diet

In columns A&B, list the nutritional facts you wish to monitor (i.e. fat, calories, sodium, sugar, protein, etc.)

| ☐ **Breakfast** | A | B |
|---|---|---|
| | | |
| | | |
| | | |
| | | |
| | | |
| Breakfast Totals | | |

| ☐ **Lunch** | | |
|---|---|---|
| | | |
| | | |
| | | |
| | | |
| | | |
| Lunch Totals | | |

| ☐ **Dinner** | | |
|---|---|---|
| | | |
| | | |
| | | |
| | | |
| | | |
| Dinner Totals | | |

| ☐ **Snacks** | | |
|---|---|---|
| | | |
| | | |
| | | |
| Snack Totals | | |

GRAND TOTALS FOR TODAY:

| A | B |
|---|---|
| | |

Memory Minder©

_____ _____
Date                    Day

| | AM | PM |
|---|---|---|
| Weight | | |
| Temperature | | |
| Blood Pressure | | |
| Sugar Level | | |
| Hours slept last night | Number of hours: | Sound ☐ Restless ☐ |
| Naps taken today | How many? | Total hours: |

## Today's Weather

☐ Hot      ☐ Sunny      ☐ Damp
☐ Warm     ☐ Cloudy     ☐ Rainy
☐ Cool     ☐ Overcast   ☐ Snowy
☐ Cold     ☐ Foggy      ☐ Windy

## Drugs / Medications

| Qty | | Description | Strength |
|---|---|---|---|
| AM | PM | | |
| | | | |
| | | | |
| | | | |
| | | | |
| | | | |
| | | | |
| | | | |

## Vitamins / Herbs

| Qty | | Description | Strength |
|---|---|---|---|
| AM | PM | | |
| | | | |
| | | | |
| | | | |
| | | | |
| | | | |
| | | | |

MemoryMinder©

## Physical Activity

| Activity | Hours | Mins. |
|---|---|---|
| | | |
| | | |
| | | |
| | | |

## Pain / Discomfort / Skin Changes

### Scale

1 Mild
2 Moderate
3 Severe
4 Very Severe
5 Worst Possible

Mark the area where the pain occurs with the number which corresponds to the intensity of the pain.

## In general, today I felt:

☐ Good
☐ Fair
☐ Poor

## Today's Conditions and Symptoms

Check the areas which apply and explain your conditions or symptoms in the space provided. See the *Symptoms Glossary* to help you describe your conditions.

☐ *Ears / Eyes / Nose*
_____

☐ *Mouth / Throat*
_____

☐ *Head / Neck / Back*
_____

☐ *Shoulders / Arms / Hands*
_____

☐ *Chest / Heart*
_____

☐ *Respiratory System*
_____

☐ *Digestive System*
_____

☐ *Hips / Legs / Feet*
_____

☐ *Male / Female Organs*
_____

☐ *Skin*
_____

☐ *Mood*
_____

☐ *Other*
_____
_____

## Comments
_____
_____
_____
_____

## Today's Diet

In columns A&B, list the nutritional facts you wish to monitor (i.e. fat, calories, sodium, sugar, protein, etc.)

| ☐ **Breakfast** | A | B |
| --- | --- | --- |
|  |  |  |
|  |  |  |
|  |  |  |
|  |  |  |
|  |  |  |
| Breakfast Totals |  |  |

| ☐ **Lunch** |  |  |
| --- | --- | --- |
|  |  |  |
|  |  |  |
|  |  |  |
|  |  |  |
|  |  |  |
| Lunch Totals |  |  |

| ☐ **Dinner** |  |  |
| --- | --- | --- |
|  |  |  |
|  |  |  |
|  |  |  |
|  |  |  |
|  |  |  |
|  |  |  |
| Dinner Totals |  |  |

| ☐ **Snacks** |  |  |
| --- | --- | --- |
|  |  |  |
|  |  |  |
|  |  |  |
| Snack Totals |  |  |

GRAND TOTALS FOR TODAY:

| A | B |
| --- | --- |
|  |  |

MemoryMinder©

_____ _____
Date                Day

## Today's Weather

| | AM | PM |
|---|---|---|
| Weight | | |
| Temperature | | |
| Blood Pressure | | |
| Sugar Level | | |
| Hours slept last night | Number of hours: | Sound ☐ Restless ☐ |
| Naps taken today | How many? | Total hours: |

### Today's Weather

- ☐ Hot
- ☐ Warm
- ☐ Cool
- ☐ Cold
- ☐ Sunny
- ☐ Cloudy
- ☐ Overcast
- ☐ Foggy
- ☐ Damp
- ☐ Rainy
- ☐ Snowy
- ☐ Windy

## Drugs / Medications

| Qty | | Description | Strength |
|---|---|---|---|
| AM | PM | | |
| | | | |
| | | | |
| | | | |
| | | | |
| | | | |
| | | | |
| | | | |

## Vitamins / Herbs

| Qty | | Description | Strength |
|---|---|---|---|
| AM | PM | | |
| | | | |
| | | | |
| | | | |
| | | | |
| | | | |
| | | | |
| | | | |

MemoryMinder©

## Physical Activity

| Activity | Hours | Mins. |
|---|---|---|
| | | |
| | | |
| | | |
| | | |

## Pain / Discomfort / Skin Changes

### Scale

1 Mild
2 Moderate
3 Severe
4 Very Severe
5 Worst Possible

Mark the area where the pain occurs with the number which corresponds to the intensity of the pain.

### In general, today I felt:

- ☐ Good
- ☐ Fair
- ☐ Poor

## Today's Conditions and Symptoms

Check the areas which apply and explain your conditions or symptoms in the space provided. See the *Symptoms Glossary* to help you describe your conditions.

☐ *Ears / Eyes / Nose*
_____
_____

☐ *Mouth / Throat*
_____
_____

☐ *Head / Neck / Back*
_____
_____

☐ *Shoulders / Arms / Hands*
_____
_____

☐ *Chest / Heart*
_____
_____

☐ *Respiratory System*
_____
_____

☐ *Digestive System*
_____
_____

☐ *Hips / Legs / Feet*
_____
_____

☐ *Male / Female Organs*
_____
_____

☐ *Skin*
_____
_____

☐ *Mood*
_____
_____

☐ *Other*
_____
_____
_____

## Comments
_____
_____
_____
_____
_____

MemoryMinder©

## Today's Diet

In columns A&B, list the nutritional facts you wish to monitor (i.e. fat, calories, sodium, sugar, protein, etc.)

☐ **Breakfast**

| | A | B |
|---|---|---|
| | | |
| | | |
| | | |
| | | |
| | | |
| Breakfast Totals | | |

☐ **Lunch**

| | A | B |
|---|---|---|
| | | |
| | | |
| | | |
| | | |
| | | |
| Lunch Totals | | |

☐ **Dinner**

| | A | B |
|---|---|---|
| | | |
| | | |
| | | |
| | | |
| | | |
| Dinner Totals | | |

☐ **Snacks**

| | A | B |
|---|---|---|
| | | |
| | | |
| | | |
| Snack Totals | | |

GRAND TOTALS FOR TODAY:

| A | B |
|---|---|
| | |

| | | AM | PM |
|---|---|---|---|
| Weight | | | |
| Temperature | | | |
| Blood Pressure | | | |
| Sugar Level | | | |
| Hours slept last night | | Number of hours: | Sound ☐ Restless ☐ |
| Naps taken today | | How many? | Total hours: |

_____ _____
Date · Day

## *Today's Weather*

☐ Hot    ☐ Sunny    ☐ Damp
☐ Warm    ☐ Cloudy    ☐ Rainy
☐ Cool    ☐ Overcast    ☐ Snowy
☐ Cold    ☐ Foggy    ☐ Windy

## *Drugs / Medications*

| Qty | | Description | Strength |
|---|---|---|---|
| AM | PM | | |
| | | | |
| | | | |
| | | | |
| | | | |
| | | | |
| | | | |

## *Vitamins / Herbs*

| Qty | | Description | Strength |
|---|---|---|---|
| AM | PM | | |
| | | | |
| | | | |
| | | | |
| | | | |
| | | | |
| | | | |

MemoryMinder©

## *Physical Activity*

| Activity | Hours | Mins. |
|---|---|---|
| | | |
| | | |
| | | |
| | | |

## *Pain / Discomfort / Skin Changes*

### Scale

1 Mild
2 Moderate
3 Severe
4 Very Severe
5 Worst Possible

Mark the area where the pain occurs with the number which corresponds to the intensity of the pain.

### *In general, today I felt:*

☐ Good

☐ Fair

☐ Poor

## Today's Conditions and Symptoms

Check the areas which apply and explain your conditions or symptoms in the space provided. See the *Symptoms Glossary* to help you describe your conditions.

☐ *Ears / Eyes / Nose*
_____

☐ *Mouth / Throat*
_____

☐ *Head / Neck / Back*
_____

☐ *Shoulders / Arms / Hands*
_____

☐ *Chest / Heart*
_____

☐ *Respiratory System*
_____

☐ *Digestive System*
_____

☐ *Hips / Legs / Feet*
_____

☐ *Male / Female Organs*
_____

☐ *Skin*
_____

☐ *Mood*
_____

☐ *Other*
_____
_____

## Comments

_____
_____
_____
_____

MemoryMinder©

## Today's Diet

In columns A&B, list the nutritional facts you wish to monitor (i.e. fat, calories, sodium, sugar, protein, etc.)

| ☐ **Breakfast** | A | B |
|---|---|---|
| | | |
| | | |
| | | |
| | | |
| | | |
| Breakfast Totals | | |

| ☐ **Lunch** | | |
|---|---|---|
| | | |
| | | |
| | | |
| | | |
| | | |
| Lunch Totals | | |

| ☐ **Dinner** | | |
|---|---|---|
| | | |
| | | |
| | | |
| | | |
| | | |
| Dinner Totals | | |

| ☐ **Snacks** | | |
|---|---|---|
| | | |
| | | |
| | | |
| Snack Totals | | |

| GRAND TOTALS FOR TODAY: | |
|---|---|
| A | B |

| | Date | | Day |
| --- | --- | --- | --- |
| _____ | | _____ | |

| | AM | PM |
| --- | --- | --- |
| Weight | | |
| Temperature | | |
| Blood Pressure | / | / |
| Sugar Level | | |
| Hours slept last night | Number of hours: | Sound ☐ Restless ☐ |
| Naps taken today | How many? | Total hours: |

## Today's Weather

☐ Hot  ☐ Sunny  ☐ Damp
☐ Warm  ☐ Cloudy  ☐ Rainy
☐ Cool  ☐ Overcast  ☐ Snowy
☐ Cold  ☐ Foggy  ☐ Windy

## Drugs / Medications

| Qty | | Description | Strength |
| --- | --- | --- | --- |
| AM | PM | | |
| | | | |
| | | | |
| | | | |
| | | | |
| | | | |
| | | | |

## Vitamins / Herbs

| Qty | | Description | Strengt* |
| --- | --- | --- | --- |
| AM | PM | | |
| | | | |
| | | | |
| | | | |
| | | | |
| | | | |
| | | | |

MemoryMinder©

## Physical Activity

| Activity | Hours | Mins. |
| --- | --- | --- |
| | | |
| | | |
| | | |

## Pain / Discomfort / Skin Changes

### Scale

1 Mild
2 Moderate
3 Severe
4 Very Severe
5 Worst Possible

Mark the area where the pain occurs with the number which corresponds to the intensity of the pain.

### In general, today I felt:

☐ Good
☐ Fair
☐ Poor

## Today's Conditions and Symptoms

Check the areas which apply and explain your conditions or symptoms in the space provided. See the *Symptoms Glossary* to help you describe your conditions.

☐ *Ears / Eyes / Nose*
_____

☐ *Mouth / Throat*
_____

☐ *Head / Neck / Back*
_____

☐ *Shoulders / Arms / Hands*
_____

☐ *Chest / Heart*
_____

☐ *Respiratory System*
_____

☐ *Digestive System*
_____

☐ *Hips / Legs / Feet*
_____

☐ *Male / Female Organs*
_____

☐ *Skin*
_____

☐ *Mood*
_____

☐ *Other*
_____
_____

## Comments
_____
_____
_____
_____

## Today's Diet

In columns A&B, list the nutritional facts you wish to monitor (i.e. fat, calories, sodium, sugar, protein, etc.)

| ☐ Breakfast | A | B |
|---|---|---|
| | | |
| | | |
| | | |
| | | |
| Breakfast Totals | | |

| ☐ Lunch | | |
|---|---|---|
| | | |
| | | |
| | | |
| | | |
| | | |
| Lunch Totals | | |

| ☐ Dinner | | |
|---|---|---|
| | | |
| | | |
| | | |
| | | |
| | | |
| Dinner Totals | | |

| ☐ Snacks | | |
|---|---|---|
| | | |
| | | |
| | | |
| Snack Totals | | |

GRAND TOTALS FOR TODAY:

| A | B |
|---|---|
| | |

MemoryMinder©

_____  _____
Date                    Day

## Today's Weather

- [ ] Hot
- [ ] Warm
- [ ] Cool
- [ ] Cold
- [ ] Sunny
- [ ] Cloudy
- [ ] Overcast
- [ ] Foggy
- [ ] Damp
- [ ] Rainy
- [ ] Snowy
- [ ] Windy

| | AM | PM |
|---|---|---|
| Weight | | |
| Temperature | | |
| Blood Pressure | | |
| Sugar Level | | |
| Hours slept last night | Number of hours: | Sound ☐ Restless ☐ |
| Naps taken today | How many? | Total hours: |

## Drugs / Medications

| Qty | | Description | Strength |
|---|---|---|---|
| AM | PM | | |
| | | | |
| | | | |
| | | | |
| | | | |
| | | | |
| | | | |

## Vitamins / Herbs

| Qty | | Description | Strength |
|---|---|---|---|
| AM | PM | | |
| | | | |
| | | | |
| | | | |
| | | | |
| | | | |

MemoryMinder©

## Physical Activity

| Activity | Hours | Mins. |
|---|---|---|
| | | |
| | | |
| | | |

## Pain / Discomfort / Skin Changes

### Scale

1 Mild
2 Moderate
3 Severe
4 Very Severe
5 Worst Possible

Mark the area where the pain occurs with the number which corresponds to the intensity of the pain.

### In general, today I felt:

- [ ] Good
- [ ] Fair
- [ ] Poor

## Today's Conditions and Symptoms

Check the areas which apply and explain your conditions or symptoms in the space provided. See the *Symptoms Glossary* to help you describe your conditions.

☐ *Ears / Eyes / Nose*
_____

☐ *Mouth / Throat*
_____

☐ *Head / Neck / Back*
_____

☐ *Shoulders / Arms / Hands*
_____

☐ *Chest / Heart*
_____

☐ *Respiratory System*
_____

☐ *Digestive System*
_____

☐ *Hips / Legs / Feet*
_____

☐ *Male / Female Organs*
_____

☐ *Skin*
_____

☐ *Mood*
_____

☐ *Other*
_____
_____

## Comments
_____
_____
_____
_____

MemoryMinder©

## Today's Diet

In columns A&B, list the nutritional facts you wish to monitor (i.e. fat, calories, sodium, sugar, protein, etc.)

| ☐ **Breakfast** | A | B |
|---|---|---|
|  |  |  |
|  |  |  |
|  |  |  |
|  |  |  |
|  |  |  |
| Breakfast Totals |  |  |

| ☐ **Lunch** | | |
|---|---|---|
|  |  |  |
|  |  |  |
|  |  |  |
|  |  |  |
|  |  |  |
|  |  |  |
| Lunch Totals |  |  |

| ☐ **Dinner** | | |
|---|---|---|
|  |  |  |
|  |  |  |
|  |  |  |
|  |  |  |
|  |  |  |
|  |  |  |
| Dinner Totals |  |  |

| ☐ **Snacks** | | |
|---|---|---|
|  |  |  |
|  |  |  |
|  |  |  |
| Snack Totals |  |  |

GRAND TOTALS FOR TODAY:

| A | B |
|---|---|
|  |  |

| | Date | | Day |
| --- | --- | --- | --- |

## Today's Weather

- [ ] Hot
- [ ] Warm
- [ ] Cool
- [ ] Cold
- [ ] Sunny
- [ ] Cloudy
- [ ] Overcast
- [ ] Foggy
- [ ] Damp
- [ ] Rainy
- [ ] Snowy
- [ ] Windy

| | AM | PM |
| --- | --- | --- |
| Weight | | |
| Temperature | | |
| Blood Pressure | | |
| Sugar Level | | |
| Hours slept last night | Number of hours: | Sound ☐ Restless ☐ |
| Naps taken today | How many? | Total hours: |

## Drugs / Medications

| Qty | | Description | Strength |
| --- | --- | --- | --- |
| AM | PM | | |
| | | | |
| | | | |
| | | | |
| | | | |
| | | | |
| | | | |

## Vitamins / Herbs

| Qty | | Description | Strength |
| --- | --- | --- | --- |
| AM | PM | | |
| | | | |
| | | | |
| | | | |
| | | | |
| | | | |

MemoryMinder©

## Physical Activity

| Activity | Hours | Mins. |
| --- | --- | --- |
| | | |
| | | |
| | | |
| | | |

## Pain / Discomfort / Skin Changes

### Scale

1 Mild
2 Moderate
3 Severe
4 Very Severe
5 Worst Possible

Mark the area where the pain occurs with the number which corresponds to the intensity of the pain.

### In general, today I felt:

- [ ] Good
- [ ] Fair
- [ ] Poor

# Today's Conditions and Symptoms

Check the areas which apply and explain your conditions or symptoms in the space provided. See the *Symptoms Glossary* to help you describe your conditions.

☐ **Ears / Eyes / Nose**

_____

☐ **Mouth / Throat**

_____

☐ **Head / Neck / Back**

_____

☐ **Shoulders / Arms / Hands**

_____

☐ **Chest / Heart**

_____

☐ **Respiratory System**

_____

☐ **Digestive System**

_____

☐ **Hips / Legs / Feet**

_____

☐ **Male / Female Organs**

_____

☐ **Skin**

_____

☐ **Mood**

_____

☐ **Other**

_____
_____

## Comments

_____
_____
_____
_____

MemoryMinder©

# Today's Diet

In columns A&B, list the nutritional facts you wish to monitor (i.e. fat, calories, sodium, sugar, protein, etc.)

| ☐ **Breakfast** | A | B |
|---|---|---|
| | | |
| | | |
| | | |
| | | |
| | | |
| Breakfast Totals | | |

| ☐ **Lunch** | | |
|---|---|---|
| | | |
| | | |
| | | |
| | | |
| | | |
| Lunch Totals | | |

| ☐ **Dinner** | | |
|---|---|---|
| | | |
| | | |
| | | |
| | | |
| | | |
| Dinner Totals | | |

| ☐ **Snacks** | | |
|---|---|---|
| | | |
| | | |
| | | |
| Snack Totals | | |

GRAND TOTALS FOR TODAY:

| A | B |
|---|---|
| | |

|  | AM | PM |
|---|---|---|
| Weight | | |
| Temperature | | |
| Blood Pressure | | |
| Sugar Level | | |

| Date | Day |
|---|---|

## Today's Weather

- [ ] Hot
- [ ] Warm
- [ ] Cool
- [ ] Cold
- [ ] Sunny
- [ ] Cloudy
- [ ] Overcast
- [ ] Foggy
- [ ] Damp
- [ ] Rainy
- [ ] Snowy
- [ ] Windy

| Hours slept last night | Number of hours: | Sound [ ] Restless [ ] |
|---|---|---|
| Naps taken today | How many? | Total hours: |

## Drugs / Medications

| Qty | | Description | Strength |
|---|---|---|---|
| AM | PM | | |
| | | | |
| | | | |
| | | | |
| | | | |
| | | | |
| | | | |

## Vitamins / Herbs

| Qty | | Description | Strength |
|---|---|---|---|
| AM | PM | | |
| | | | |
| | | | |
| | | | |
| | | | |
| | | | |
| | | | |

MemoryMinder©

## Physical Activity

| Activity | Hours | Mins. |
|---|---|---|
| | | |
| | | |
| | | |
| | | |

## Pain / Discomfort / Skin Changes

### Scale

1 Mild
2 Moderate
3 Severe
4 Very Severe
5 Worst Possible

Mark the area where the pain occurs with the number which corresponds to the intensity of the pain.

### In general, today I felt:

- [ ] Good
- [ ] Fair
- [ ] Poor

# Today's Conditions and Symptoms

Check the areas which apply and explain your conditions or symptoms in the space provided. See the *Symptoms Glossary* to help you describe your conditions.

☐ **Ears / Eyes / Nose**
_____

☐ **Mouth / Throat**
_____

☐ **Head / Neck / Back**
_____

☐ **Shoulders / Arms / Hands**
_____

☐ **Chest / Heart**
_____

☐ **Respiratory System**
_____

☐ **Digestive System**
_____

☐ **Hips / Legs / Feet**
_____

☐ **Male / Female Organs**
_____

☐ **Skin**
_____

☐ **Mood**
_____

☐ **Other**
_____
_____

# Comments

_____
_____
_____
_____

MemoryMinder©

# Today's Diet

In columns A&B, list the nutritional facts you wish to monitor (i.e. fat, calories, sodium, sugar, protein, etc.)

☐ **Breakfast**    A    B

Breakfast Totals

☐ **Lunch**

Lunch Totals

☐ **Dinner**

Dinner Totals

☐ **Snacks**

Snack Totals

GRAND TOTALS FOR TODAY:

A _____    B _____

| | Date | | Day | | AM | PM |
|---|---|---|---|---|---|---|

| | AM | PM |
|---|---|---|
| Weight | | |
| Temperature | | |
| Blood Pressure | | |
| Sugar Level | | |
| Hours slept last night | Number of hours: | Sound / Restless |
| Naps taken today | How many? | Total hours: |

_____   _____
Date                        Day

## Today's Weather

- ☐ Hot
- ☐ Warm
- ☐ Cool
- ☐ Cold
- ☐ Sunny
- ☐ Cloudy
- ☐ Overcast
- ☐ Foggy
- ☐ Damp
- ☐ Rainy
- ☐ Snowy
- ☐ Windy

## Drugs / Medications

| Qty | | Description | Strength |
|---|---|---|---|
| AM | PM | | |
| | | | |
| | | | |
| | | | |
| | | | |
| | | | |
| | | | |

## Vitamins / Herbs

| Qty | | Description | Strength |
|---|---|---|---|
| AM | PM | | |
| | | | |
| | | | |
| | | | |
| | | | |
| | | | |
| | | | |

MemoryMinder©

## Physical Activity

| Activity | Hours | Mins. |
|---|---|---|
| | | |
| | | |
| | | |

## Pain / Discomfort / Skin Changes

### Scale

1 Mild
2 Moderate
3 Severe
4 Very Severe
5 Worst Possible

Mark the area where the pain occurs with the number which corresponds to the intensity of the pain.

### In general, today I felt:

- ☐ Good
- ☐ Fair
- ☐ Poor

## Today's Conditions and Symptoms

Check the areas which apply and explain your conditions or symptoms in the space provided. See the *Symptoms Glossary* to help you describe your conditions.

☐ *Ears / Eyes / Nose*
_____
_____

☐ *Mouth / Throat*
_____
_____

☐ *Head / Neck / Back*
_____
_____

☐ *Shoulders / Arms / Hands*
_____
_____

☐ *Chest / Heart*
_____
_____

☐ *Respiratory System*
_____
_____

☐ *Digestive System*
_____
_____

☐ *Hips / Legs / Feet*
_____
_____

☐ *Male / Female Organs*
_____
_____

☐ *Skin*
_____
_____

☐ *Mood*
_____
_____

☐ *Other*
_____
_____
_____

### Comments
_____
_____
_____
_____

## Today's Diet

In columns A&B, list the nutritional facts you wish to monitor (i.e. fat, calories, sodium, sugar, protein, etc.)

☐ **Breakfast**

| | A | B |
|---|---|---|
| | | |
| | | |
| | | |
| | | |
| | | |
| Breakfast Totals | | |

☐ **Lunch**

| | | |
|---|---|---|
| | | |
| | | |
| | | |
| | | |
| | | |
| Lunch Totals | | |

☐ **Dinner**

| | | |
|---|---|---|
| | | |
| | | |
| | | |
| | | |
| | | |
| | | |
| Dinner Totals | | |

☐ **Snacks**

| | | |
|---|---|---|
| | | |
| | | |
| | | |
| Snack Totals | | |

GRAND TOTALS FOR TODAY:

| A | B |
|---|---|
| | |

MemoryMinder©

| | Date | | Day | |
|---|---|---|---|---|

## Today's Weather

| | | |
|---|---|---|
| ☐ Hot | ☐ Sunny | ☐ Damp |
| ☐ Warm | ☐ Cloudy | ☐ Rainy |
| ☐ Cool | ☐ Overcast | ☐ Snowy |
| ☐ Cold | ☐ Foggy | ☐ Windy |

| | AM | PM |
|---|---|---|
| Weight | | |
| Temperature | | |
| Blood Pressure | | |
| Sugar Level | | |
| Hours slept last night | Number of hours: | Sound ☐ Restless ☐ |
| Naps taken today | How many? | Total hours: |

## Drugs / Medications

| Qty | | Description | Strength |
|---|---|---|---|
| AM | PM | | |
| | | | |
| | | | |
| | | | |
| | | | |
| | | | |
| | | | |

## Vitamins / Herbs

| Qty | | Description | Strength |
|---|---|---|---|
| AM | PM | | |
| | | | |
| | | | |
| | | | |
| | | | |
| | | | |
| | | | |

MemoryMinder©

## Physical Activity

| Activity | Hours | Mins. |
|---|---|---|
| | | |
| | | |
| | | |

## Pain / Discomfort / Skin Changes

### Scale

1 Mild
2 Moderate
3 Severe
4 Very Severe
5 Worst Possible

Mark the area where the pain occurs with the number which corresponds to the intensity of the pain.

### In general, today I felt:

☐ Good
☐ Fair
☐ Poor

# Today's Conditions and Symptoms

Check the areas which apply and explain your conditions or symptoms in the space provided. See the *Symptoms Glossary* to help you describe your conditions.

☐ *Ears / Eyes / Nose*

_____

☐ *Mouth / Throat*

_____

☐ *Head / Neck / Back*

_____

☐ *Shoulders / Arms / Hands*

_____

☐ *Chest / Heart*

_____

☐ *Respiratory System*

_____

☐ *Digestive System*

_____

☐ *Hips / Legs / Feet*

_____

☐ *Male / Female Organs*

_____

☐ *Skin*

_____

☐ *Mood*

_____

☐ *Other*

_____

_____

## Comments

_____
_____
_____
_____

MemoryMinder©

# Today's Diet

In columns A&B, list the nutritional facts you wish to monitor (i.e. fat, calories, sodium, sugar, protein, etc.)

☐ **Breakfast**

| | A | B |
|---|---|---|
| | | |
| | | |
| | | |
| | | |
| | | |
| Breakfast Totals | | |

☐ **Lunch**

| | | |
|---|---|---|
| | | |
| | | |
| | | |
| | | |
| | | |
| Lunch Totals | | |

☐ **Dinner**

| | | |
|---|---|---|
| | | |
| | | |
| | | |
| | | |
| | | |
| Dinner Totals | | |

☐ **Snacks**

| | | |
|---|---|---|
| | | |
| | | |
| | | |
| Snack Totals | | |

GRAND TOTALS FOR TODAY:

| A | B |
|---|---|
| | |

|  | Date | Day |
|--|------|-----|

## Today's Weather

| | | |
|--|--|--|
| ☐ Hot | ☐ Sunny | ☐ Damp |
| ☐ Warm | ☐ Cloudy | ☐ Rainy |
| ☐ Cool | ☐ Overcast | ☐ Snowy |
| ☐ Cold | ☐ Foggy | ☐ Windy |

|  | AM | PM |
|--|----|----|
| Weight | | |
| Temperature | | |
| Blood Pressure | | |
| Sugar Level | | |
| Hours slept last night | Number of hours: | Sound ☐ Restless ☐ |
| Naps taken today | How many? | Total hours: |

## Drugs / Medications

| Qty | | Description | Strength |
|-----|-----|-------------|----------|
| AM | PM | | |
| | | | |
| | | | |
| | | | |
| | | | |
| | | | |
| | | | |
| | | | |

## Vitamins / Herbs

| Qty | | Description | Strength |
|-----|-----|-------------|----------|
| AM | PM | | |
| | | | |
| | | | |
| | | | |
| | | | |
| | | | |
| | | | |

MemoryMinder©

## Physical Activity

| Activity | Hours | Mins. |
|----------|-------|-------|
| | | |
| | | |
| | | |
| | | |

## Pain / Discomfort / Skin Changes

### Scale

1 Mild
2 Moderate
3 Severe
4 Very Severe
5 Worst Possible

Mark the area where the pain occurs with the number which corresponds to the intensity of the pain.

### In general, today I felt:

☐ Good

☐ Fair

☐ Poor

## Today's Conditions and Symptoms

Check the areas which apply and explain your conditions or symptoms in the space provided. See the *Symptoms Glossary* to help you describe your conditions.

☐ *Ears / Eyes / Nose*

_____

☐ *Mouth / Throat*

_____

☐ *Head / Neck / Back*

_____

☐ *Shoulders / Arms / Hands*

_____

☐ *Chest / Heart*

_____

☐ *Respiratory System*

_____

☐ *Digestive System*

_____

☐ *Hips / Legs / Feet*

_____

☐ *Male / Female Organs*

_____

☐ *Skin*

_____

☐ *Mood*

_____

☐ *Other*

_____

## Comments

_____
_____
_____
_____

## Today's Diet

In columns A&B, list the nutritional facts you wish to monitor (i.e. fat, calories, sodium, sugar, protein, etc.)

| ☐ **Breakfast** | A | B |
|---|---|---|
| | | |
| | | |
| | | |
| | | |
| Breakfast Totals | | |

| ☐ **Lunch** | | |
|---|---|---|
| | | |
| | | |
| | | |
| | | |
| Lunch Totals | | |

| ☐ **Dinner** | | |
|---|---|---|
| | | |
| | | |
| | | |
| | | |
| Dinner Totals | | |

| ☐ **Snacks** | | |
|---|---|---|
| | | |
| | | |
| Snack Totals | | |

GRAND TOTALS FOR TODAY:

| A | B |
|---|---|
| | |

MemoryMinder©

| | Date | | Day |
| --- | --- | --- | --- |

| | AM | PM |
| --- | --- | --- |
| Weight | | |
| Temperature | | |
| Blood Pressure | | |
| Sugar Level | | |
| Hours slept last night | Number of hours: | Sound ☐ Restless ☐ |
| Naps taken today | How many? | Total hours: |

## Today's Weather

☐ Hot  ☐ Sunny  ☐ Damp
☐ Warm  ☐ Cloudy  ☐ Rainy
☐ Cool  ☐ Overcast  ☐ Snowy
☐ Cold  ☐ Foggy  ☐ Windy

## Drugs / Medications

| Qty | | Description | Strength |
| --- | --- | --- | --- |
| AM | PM | | |
| | | | |
| | | | |
| | | | |
| | | | |
| | | | |
| | | | |

## Vitamins / Herbs

| Qty | | Description | Strength |
| --- | --- | --- | --- |
| AM | PM | | |
| | | | |
| | | | |
| | | | |
| | | | |
| | | | |
| | | | |

MemoryMinder©

## Physical Activity

| Activity | Hours | Mins. |
| --- | --- | --- |
| | | |
| | | |
| | | |

## Pain / Discomfort / Skin Changes

### Scale

1 Mild
2 Moderate
3 Severe
4 Very Severe
5 Worst Possible

Mark the area where the pain occurs with the number which corresponds to the intensity of the pain.

### In general, today I felt:

☐ Good
☐ Fair
☐ Poor

## Today's Conditions and Symptoms

Check the areas which apply and explain your conditions or symptoms in the space provided. See the *Symptoms Glossary* to help you describe your conditions.

☐ *Ears / Eyes / Nose*

_____

_____

☐ *Mouth / Throat*

_____

_____

☐ *Head / Neck / Back*

_____

_____

☐ *Shoulders / Arms / Hands*

_____

_____

☐ *Chest / Heart*

_____

_____

☐ *Respiratory System*

_____

_____

☐ *Digestive System*

_____

_____

☐ *Hips / Legs / Feet*

_____

_____

☐ *Male / Female Organs*

_____

_____

☐ *Skin*

_____

_____

☐ *Mood*

_____

_____

☐ *Other*

_____

_____

_____

## Comments

_____

_____

_____

_____

MemoryMinder©

## Today's Diet

In columns A&B, list the nutritional facts you wish to monitor (i.e. fat, calories, sodium, sugar, protein, etc.)

☐ **Breakfast**

| | A | B |
|---|---|---|
| | | |
| | | |
| | | |
| | | |
| Breakfast Totals | | |

☐ **Lunch**

| | A | B |
|---|---|---|
| | | |
| | | |
| | | |
| | | |
| Lunch Totals | | |

☐ **Dinner**

| | A | B |
|---|---|---|
| | | |
| | | |
| | | |
| | | |
| Dinner Totals | | |

☐ **Snacks**

| | A | B |
|---|---|---|
| | | |
| | | |
| Snack Totals | | |

GRAND TOTALS FOR TODAY:

| A | B |
|---|---|
| | |

| | AM | PM |
|---|---|---|
| _____ _____ | | |
| Date          Day | | |

## *Today's Weather*

| | AM | PM |
|---|---|---|
| Weight | | |
| Temperature | | |
| Blood Pressure | | |
| Sugar Level | | |
| Hours slept last night | Number of hours: | Sound ☐ Restless ☐ |
| Naps taken today | How many? | Total hours: |

**Today's Weather**

- ☐ Hot
- ☐ Warm
- ☐ Cool
- ☐ Cold
- ☐ Sunny
- ☐ Cloudy
- ☐ Overcast
- ☐ Foggy
- ☐ Damp
- ☐ Rainy
- ☐ Snowy
- ☐ Windy

## *Drugs / Medications*

| Qty | | Description | Strength |
|---|---|---|---|
| AM | PM | | |
| | | | |
| | | | |
| | | | |
| | | | |
| | | | |
| | | | |
| | | | |

## *Vitamins / Herbs*

| Qty | | Description | Strengt |
|---|---|---|---|
| AM | PM | | |
| | | | |
| | | | |
| | | | |
| | | | |
| | | | |
| | | | |

MemoryMinder©

## *Physical Activity*

| Activity | Hours | Mins. |
|---|---|---|
| | | |
| | | |
| | | |

## *Pain / Discomfort / Skin Changes*

### Scale

1 Mild
2 Moderate
3 Severe
4 Very Severe
5 Worst Possible

Mark the area where the pain occurs with the number which corresponds to the intensity of the pain.

### *In general, today I felt:*

- ☐ Good
- ☐ Fair
- ☐ Poor

## Today's Conditions and Symptoms

Check the areas which apply and explain your conditions or symptoms in the space provided. See the *Symptoms Glossary* to help you describe your conditions.

☐ *Ears / Eyes / Nose*

_____

☐ *Mouth / Throat*

_____

☐ *Head / Neck / Back*

_____

☐ *Shoulders / Arms / Hands*

_____

☐ *Chest / Heart*

_____

☐ *Respiratory System*

_____

☐ *Digestive System*

_____

☐ *Hips / Legs / Feet*

_____

☐ *Male / Female Organs*

_____

☐ *Skin*

_____

☐ *Mood*

_____

☐ *Other*

_____
_____

## Comments

_____
_____
_____
_____

MemoryMinder©

## Today's Diet

In columns A&B, list the nutritional facts you wish to monitor (i.e. fat, calories, sodium, sugar, protein, etc.)

☐ *Breakfast*

| | A | B |
|---|---|---|
| | | |
| | | |
| | | |
| | | |
| Breakfast Totals | | |

☐ *Lunch*

| | A | B |
|---|---|---|
| | | |
| | | |
| | | |
| | | |
| Lunch Totals | | |

☐ *Dinner*

| | A | B |
|---|---|---|
| | | |
| | | |
| | | |
| | | |
| Dinner Totals | | |

☐ *Snacks*

| | A | B |
|---|---|---|
| | | |
| | | |
| Snack Totals | | |

GRAND TOTALS FOR TODAY:

| A | B |
|---|---|
| | |

| | Date | Day |
|---|---|---|

## Today's Weather

- [ ] Hot
- [ ] Warm
- [ ] Cool
- [ ] Cold
- [ ] Sunny
- [ ] Cloudy
- [ ] Overcast
- [ ] Foggy
- [ ] Damp
- [ ] Rainy
- [ ] Snowy
- [ ] Windy

| | AM | PM |
|---|---|---|
| Weight | | |
| Temperature | | |
| Blood Pressure | | |
| Sugar Level | | |
| Hours slept last night | Number of hours: | Sound ☐ Restless ☐ |
| Naps taken today | How many? | Total hours: |

## Drugs / Medications

| Qty | | Description | Strength |
|---|---|---|---|
| AM | PM | | |
| | | | |
| | | | |
| | | | |
| | | | |
| | | | |
| | | | |

## Vitamins / Herbs

| Qty | | Description | Strengt* |
|---|---|---|---|
| AM | PM | | |
| | | | |
| | | | |
| | | | |
| | | | |
| | | | |
| | | | |

MemoryMinder©

## Physical Activity

| Activity | Hours | Mins. |
|---|---|---|
| | | |
| | | |
| | | |
| | | |

## Pain / Discomfort / Skin Changes

### Scale

1 Mild
2 Moderate
3 Severe
4 Very Severe
5 Worst Possible

Mark the area where the pain occurs with the number which corresponds to the intensity of the pain.

### In general, today I felt:

- [ ] Good
- [ ] Fair
- [ ] Poor

# Today's Conditions and Symptoms

Check the areas which apply and explain your conditions or symptoms in the space provided. See the *Symptoms Glossary* to help you describe your conditions.

☐ *Ears / Eyes / Nose*
_____

☐ *Mouth / Throat*
_____

☐ *Head / Neck / Back*
_____

☐ *Shoulders / Arms / Hands*
_____

☐ *Chest / Heart*
_____

☐ *Respiratory System*
_____

☐ *Digestive System*
_____

☐ *Hips / Legs / Feet*
_____

☐ *Male / Female Organs*
_____

☐ *Skin*
_____

☐ *Mood*
_____

☐ *Other*
_____
_____

# Comments
_____
_____
_____
_____

# Today's Diet

In columns A&B, list the nutritional facts you wish to monitor (i.e. fat, calories, sodium, sugar, protein, etc.)

| ☐ **Breakfast** | A | B |
|---|---|---|
| | | |
| | | |
| | | |
| | | |
| | | |
| Breakfast Totals | | |

| ☐ **Lunch** | | |
|---|---|---|
| | | |
| | | |
| | | |
| | | |
| | | |
| Lunch Totals | | |

| ☐ **Dinner** | | |
|---|---|---|
| | | |
| | | |
| | | |
| | | |
| | | |
| Dinner Totals | | |

| ☐ **Snacks** | | |
|---|---|---|
| | | |
| | | |
| | | |
| Snack Totals | | |

GRAND TOTALS FOR TODAY:

| A | B |
|---|---|
| | |

MemoryMinder©

|  | AM | PM |
|---|---|---|
| Weight | | |
| Temperature | | |
| Blood Pressure | | |
| Sugar Level | | |
| Hours slept last night | Number of hours: | Sound ☐ Restless ☐ |
| Naps taken today | How many? | Total hours: |

_____ _____
Date          Day

## Today's Weather

☐ Hot  ☐ Sunny  ☐ Damp
☐ Warm  ☐ Cloudy  ☐ Rainy
☐ Cool  ☐ Overcast  ☐ Snowy
☐ Cold  ☐ Foggy  ☐ Windy

## Drugs / Medications

| Qty | | Description | Strength |
|---|---|---|---|
| AM | PM | | |
| | | | |
| | | | |
| | | | |
| | | | |
| | | | |
| | | | |

## Vitamins / Herbs

| Qty | | Description | Strength |
|---|---|---|---|
| AM | PM | | |
| | | | |
| | | | |
| | | | |
| | | | |
| | | | |
| | | | |

MemoryMinder©

## Physical Activity

| Activity | Hours | Mins. |
|---|---|---|
| | | |
| | | |
| | | |

## Pain / Discomfort / Skin Changes

### Scale

1 Mild
2 Moderate
3 Severe
4 Very Severe
5 Worst Possible

Mark the area where the pain occurs with the number which corresponds to the intensity of the pain.

### In general, today I felt:

☐ Good
☐ Fair
☐ Poor

## Today's Conditions and Symptoms

Check the areas which apply and explain your conditions or symptoms in the space provided. See the *Symptoms Glossary* to help you describe your conditions.

☐ *Ears / Eyes / Nose*

_____

☐ *Mouth / Throat*

_____

☐ *Head / Neck / Back*

_____

☐ *Shoulders / Arms / Hands*

_____

☐ *Chest / Heart*

_____

☐ *Respiratory System*

_____

☐ *Digestive System*

_____

☐ *Hips / Legs / Feet*

_____

☐ *Male / Female Organs*

_____

☐ *Skin*

_____

☐ *Mood*

_____

☐ *Other*

_____

_____

## Comments

_____
_____
_____
_____
_____

MemoryMinder©

## Today's Diet

In columns A&B, list the nutritional facts you wish to monitor (i.e. fat, calories, sodium, sugar, protein, etc.)

| ☐ **Breakfast** | A | B |
|---|---|---|
| | | |
| | | |
| | | |
| | | |
| | | |
| Breakfast Totals | | |

| ☐ **Lunch** | | |
|---|---|---|
| | | |
| | | |
| | | |
| | | |
| | | |
| Lunch Totals | | |

| ☐ **Dinner** | | |
|---|---|---|
| | | |
| | | |
| | | |
| | | |
| | | |
| Dinner Totals | | |

| ☐ **Snacks** | | |
|---|---|---|
| | | |
| | | |
| | | |
| Snack Totals | | |

GRAND TOTALS FOR TODAY:

| A | B |
|---|---|
| | |

_____ _____
Date          Day

|  | AM | PM |
|---|---|---|
| Weight | | |
| Temperature | | |
| Blood Pressure | | |
| Sugar Level | | |
| Hours slept last night | Number of hours: | Sound ☐ Restless ☐ |
| Naps taken today | How many? | Total hours: |

## Today's Weather

☐ Hot    ☐ Sunny    ☐ Damp
☐ Warm   ☐ Cloudy   ☐ Rainy
☐ Cool   ☐ Overcast ☐ Snowy
☐ Cold   ☐ Foggy    ☐ Windy

## Drugs / Medications

| Qty | | Description | Strength |
|---|---|---|---|
| AM | PM | | |
| | | | |
| | | | |
| | | | |
| | | | |
| | | | |
| | | | |

## Vitamins / Herbs

| Qty | | Description | Strengt |
|---|---|---|---|
| AM | PM | | |
| | | | |
| | | | |
| | | | |
| | | | |
| | | | |

MemoryMinder©

## Physical Activity

| Activity | Hours | Mins. |
|---|---|---|
| | | |
| | | |
| | | |

## Pain / Discomfort / Skin Changes

### Scale
1 Mild
2 Moderate
3 Severe
4 Very Severe
5 Worst Possible

Mark the area where the pain occurs with the number which corresponds to the intensity of the pain.

### In general, today I felt:

☐ Good
☐ Fair
☐ Poor

## Today's Conditions and Symptoms

Check the areas which apply and explain your conditions or symptoms in the space provided. See the *Symptoms Glossary* to help you describe your conditions.

☐ *Ears / Eyes / Nose*

_____

☐ *Mouth / Throat*

_____

☐ *Head / Neck / Back*

_____

☐ *Shoulders / Arms / Hands*

_____

☐ *Chest / Heart*

_____

☐ *Respiratory System*

_____

☐ *Digestive System*

_____

☐ *Hips / Legs / Feet*

_____

☐ *Male / Female Organs*

_____

☐ *Skin*

_____

☐ *Mood*

_____

☐ *Other*

_____

## Comments

_____
_____
_____
_____

## Today's Diet

In columns A&B, list the nutritional facts you wish to monitor (i.e. fat, calories, sodium, sugar, protein, etc.)

| ☐ **Breakfast** | A | B |
|---|---|---|
| | | |
| | | |
| | | |
| | | |
| Breakfast Totals | | |

| ☐ **Lunch** | | |
|---|---|---|
| | | |
| | | |
| | | |
| | | |
| Lunch Totals | | |

| ☐ **Dinner** | | |
|---|---|---|
| | | |
| | | |
| | | |
| | | |
| Dinner Totals | | |

| ☐ **Snacks** | | |
|---|---|---|
| | | |
| | | |
| | | |
| Snack Totals | | |

GRAND TOTALS FOR TODAY:

| A | B |
|---|---|
| | |

MemoryMinder©

_____  _____
Date                    Day

|  | AM | PM |
|---|---|---|
| Weight | | |
| Temperature | | |
| Blood Pressure | | |
| Sugar Level | | |
| Hours slept last night | Number of hours: | Sound ☐ Restless ☐ |
| Naps taken today | How many? | Total hours: |

## Today's Weather

☐ Hot        ☐ Sunny        ☐ Damp
☐ Warm       ☐ Cloudy       ☐ Rainy
☐ Cool       ☐ Overcast     ☐ Snowy
☐ Cold       ☐ Foggy        ☐ Windy

## Drugs / Medications

| Qty | | Description | Strength |
|---|---|---|---|
| AM | PM | | |
| | | | |
| | | | |
| | | | |
| | | | |
| | | | |
| | | | |

## Vitamins / Herbs

| Qty | | Description | Strength |
|---|---|---|---|
| AM | PM | | |
| | | | |
| | | | |
| | | | |
| | | | |
| | | | |
| | | | |

MemoryMinder©

## Physical Activity

| Activity | Hours | Mins. |
|---|---|---|
| | | |
| | | |
| | | |

## Pain / Discomfort / Skin Changes

### Scale

1 Mild
2 Moderate
3 Severe
4 Very Severe
5 Worst Possible

Mark the area where the pain occurs with the number which corresponds to the intensity of the pain.

### In general, today I felt:

☐ Good
☐ Fair
☐ Poor

## Today's Conditions and Symptoms

Check the areas which apply and explain your conditions or symptoms in the space provided. See the *Symptoms Glossary* to help you describe your conditions.

☐ *Ears / Eyes / Nose*

_____

☐ *Mouth / Throat*

_____

☐ *Head / Neck / Back*

_____

☐ *Shoulders / Arms / Hands*

_____

☐ *Chest / Heart*

_____

☐ *Respiratory System*

_____

☐ *Digestive System*

_____

☐ *Hips / Legs / Feet*

_____

☐ *Male / Female Organs*

_____

☐ *Skin*

_____

☐ *Mood*

_____

☐ *Other*

_____
_____

## Comments

_____
_____
_____
_____

MemoryMinder©

## Today's Diet

In columns A&B, list the nutritional facts you wish to monitor (i.e. fat, calories, sodium, sugar, protein, etc.)

| ☐ **Breakfast** | A | B |
|---|---|---|
| | | |
| | | |
| | | |
| | | |
| | | |
| Breakfast Totals | | |

| ☐ **Lunch** | | |
|---|---|---|
| | | |
| | | |
| | | |
| | | |
| | | |
| Lunch Totals | | |

| ☐ **Dinner** | | |
|---|---|---|
| | | |
| | | |
| | | |
| | | |
| | | |
| Dinner Totals | | |

| ☐ **Snacks** | | |
|---|---|---|
| | | |
| | | |
| | | |
| Snack Totals | | |

GRAND TOTALS FOR TODAY:

| A | B |
|---|---|
| | |

_____ _____
Date                     Day

| | AM | PM |
|---|---|---|
| Weight | | |
| Temperature | | |
| Blood Pressure | | |
| Sugar Level | | |
| Hours slept last night | Number of hours: | Sound ☐ Restless ☐ |
| Naps taken today | How many? | Total hours: |

## *Today's Weather*

☐ Hot      ☐ Sunny      ☐ Damp
☐ Warm    ☐ Cloudy     ☐ Rainy
☐ Cool     ☐ Overcast   ☐ Snowy
☐ Cold     ☐ Foggy      ☐ Windy

## *Drugs / Medications*

| Qty | | Description | Strength |
|---|---|---|---|
| AM | PM | | |
| | | | |
| | | | |
| | | | |
| | | | |
| | | | |
| | | | |

## *Vitamins / Herbs*

| Qty | | Description | Strength |
|---|---|---|---|
| AM | PM | | |
| | | | |
| | | | |
| | | | |
| | | | |
| | | | |
| | | | |

MemoryMinder©

## *Physical Activity*

| Activity | Hours | Mins. |
|---|---|---|
| | | |
| | | |
| | | |

## *Pain / Discomfort / Skin Changes*

### Scale

1 Mild
2 Moderate
3 Severe
4 Very Severe
5 Worst Possible

Mark the area where the pain occurs with the number which corresponds to the intensity of the pain.

### *In general, today I felt:*

☐ Good

☐ Fair

☐ Poor

# oday's Conditions and Symptoms

eck the areas which apply and explain your conditions
symptoms in the space provided. See the *Symptoms*
*ossary* to help you describe your conditions.

☐ *Ears / Eyes / Nose*
_____

☐ *Mouth / Throat*
_____

☐ *Head / Neck / Back*
_____

☐ *Shoulders / Arms / Hands*
_____

☐ *Chest / Heart*
_____

☐ *Respiratory System*
_____

☐ *Digestive System*
_____

☐ *Hips / Legs / Feet*
_____

☐ *Male / Female Organs*
_____

☐ *Skin*
_____

☐ *Mood*
_____

☐ *Other*
_____
_____

## omments
_____
_____
_____
_____

MemoryMinder©

## Today's Diet

In columns A&B, list the nutritional
facts you wish to monitor (i.e. fat,
calories, sodium, sugar, protein, etc.)

☐ **Breakfast**

| | A | B |
|---|---|---|
| | | |
| | | |
| | | |
| | | |
| | | |
| Breakfast Totals | | |

☐ **Lunch**

| | | |
|---|---|---|
| | | |
| | | |
| | | |
| | | |
| Lunch Totals | | |

☐ **Dinner**

| | | |
|---|---|---|
| | | |
| | | |
| | | |
| | | |
| | | |
| Dinner Totals | | |

☐ **Snacks**

| | | |
|---|---|---|
| | | |
| | | |
| Snack Totals | | |

GRAND TOTALS FOR TODAY:

| A | B |
|---|---|
| | |

_____  _____
Date              Day

| | | AM | PM |
|---|---|---|---|
| Weight | | | |
| Temperature | | | |
| Blood Pressure | | | |
| Sugar Level | | | |
| Hours slept last night | Number of hours: | | Sound ☐ Restless ☐ |
| Naps taken today | How many? | | Total hours: |

## Today's Weather

☐ Hot      ☐ Sunny      ☐ Damp
☐ Warm     ☐ Cloudy     ☐ Rainy
☐ Cool     ☐ Overcast   ☐ Snowy
☐ Cold     ☐ Foggy      ☐ Windy

## Drugs / Medications

| Qty | | Description | Strength |
|---|---|---|---|
| AM | PM | | |
| | | | |
| | | | |
| | | | |
| | | | |
| | | | |
| | | | |

## Vitamins / Herbs

| Qty | | Description | Streng |
|---|---|---|---|
| AM | PM | | |
| | | | |
| | | | |
| | | | |
| | | | |
| | | | |
| | | | |

MemoryMinder©

## Physical Activity

| Activity | Hours | Mins |
|---|---|---|
| | | |
| | | |
| | | |
| | | |

## Pain / Discomfort / Skin Changes

### Scale

1  Mild
2  Moderate
3  Severe
4  Very Severe
5  Worst Possible

Mark the area where the pain occurs with the number which corresponds to the intensity of the pain.

### In general, today I felt:

☐ Good
☐ Fair
☐ Poor

## Today's Conditions and Symptoms

Check the areas which apply and explain your conditions symptoms in the space provided. See the *Symptoms Glossary* to help you describe your conditions.

☐ *Ears / Eyes / Nose*
_____
_____

☐ *Mouth / Throat*
_____
_____

☐ *Head / Neck / Back*
_____
_____

☐ *Shoulders / Arms / Hands*
_____
_____

☐ *Chest / Heart*
_____
_____

☐ *Respiratory System*
_____
_____

☐ *Digestive System*
_____
_____

☐ *Hips / Legs / Feet*
_____
_____

☐ *Male / Female Organs*
_____
_____

☐ *Skin*
_____
_____

☐ *Mood*
_____
_____

☐ *Other*
_____
_____

## Comments
_____
_____
_____
_____

## Today's Diet

In columns A&B, list the nutritional facts you wish to monitor (i.e. fat, calories, sodium, sugar, protein, etc.)

| ☐ *Breakfast* | A | B |
|---|---|---|
| | | |
| | | |
| | | |
| | | |
| | | |
| Breakfast Totals | | |

| ☐ *Lunch* | | |
|---|---|---|
| | | |
| | | |
| | | |
| | | |
| | | |
| Lunch Totals | | |

| ☐ *Dinner* | | |
|---|---|---|
| | | |
| | | |
| | | |
| | | |
| | | |
| Dinner Totals | | |

| ☐ *Snacks* | | |
|---|---|---|
| | | |
| | | |
| Snack Totals | | |

GRAND TOTALS FOR TODAY:

| A | B |
|---|---|
| | |

MemoryMinder©

| | | AM | PM |
|---|---|---|---|
| _____ _____ | Weight | | |
| Date          Day | Temperature | | |
| | Blood Pressure | / | / |
| | Sugar Level | | |
| | Hours slept last night | Number of hours: | Sound ☐ Restless ☐ |
| | Naps taken today | How many? | Total hours: |

## Today's Weather

☐ Hot      ☐ Sunny      ☐ Damp
☐ Warm     ☐ Cloudy     ☐ Rainy
☐ Cool     ☐ Overcast   ☐ Snowy
☐ Cold     ☐ Foggy      ☐ Windy

## Drugs / Medications

| Qty | | Description | Strength |
|---|---|---|---|
| AM | PM | | |
| | | | |
| | | | |
| | | | |
| | | | |
| | | | |
| | | | |

## Vitamins / Herbs

| Qty | | Description | Strengt |
|---|---|---|---|
| AM | PM | | |
| | | | |
| | | | |
| | | | |
| | | | |
| | | | |
| | | | |

MemoryMinder©

## Physical Activity

| Activity | Hours | Mins. |
|---|---|---|
| | | |
| | | |
| | | |

## Pain / Discomfort / Skin Changes

### Scale

1 Mild
2 Moderate
3 Severe
4 Very Severe
5 Worst Possible

Mark the area where the pain occurs with the number which corresponds to the intensity of the pain.

### In general, today I felt:

☐ Good
☐ Fair
☐ Poor

# Today's Conditions and Symptoms

Check the areas which apply and explain your conditions or symptoms in the space provided. See the *Symptoms Glossary* to help you describe your conditions.

☐ *Ears / Eyes / Nose*
_____
_____

☐ *Mouth / Throat*
_____
_____

☐ *Head / Neck / Back*
_____
_____

☐ *Shoulders / Arms / Hands*
_____
_____

☐ *Chest / Heart*
_____
_____

☐ *Respiratory System*
_____
_____

☐ *Digestive System*
_____
_____

☐ *Hips / Legs / Feet*
_____
_____

☐ *Male / Female Organs*
_____
_____

☐ *Skin*
_____
_____

☐ *Mood*
_____
_____

☐ *Other*
_____
_____

## Comments
_____
_____
_____
_____

# Today's Diet

In columns A&B, list the nutritional facts you wish to monitor (i.e. fat, calories, sodium, sugar, protein, etc.)

| ☐ **Breakfast** | A | B |
|---|---|---|
| | | |
| | | |
| | | |
| | | |
| | | |
| Breakfast Totals | | |

| ☐ **Lunch** | | |
|---|---|---|
| | | |
| | | |
| | | |
| | | |
| | | |
| Lunch Totals | | |

| ☐ **Dinner** | | |
|---|---|---|
| | | |
| | | |
| | | |
| | | |
| | | |
| Dinner Totals | | |

| ☐ **Snacks** | | |
|---|---|---|
| | | |
| | | |
| | | |
| Snack Totals | | |

GRAND TOTALS FOR TODAY:

| A | B |
|---|---|
| | |

MemoryMinder©

| | AM | PM |
|---|---|---|
| Weight | | |
| Temperature | | |
| Blood Pressure | | |
| Sugar Level | | |
| Hours slept last night | Number of hours: | Sound ☐ Restless ☐ |
| Naps taken today | How many? | Total hours: |

## Today's Weather

☐ Hot     ☐ Sunny     ☐ Damp
☐ Warm    ☐ Cloudy    ☐ Rainy
☐ Cool    ☐ Overcast  ☐ Snowy
☐ Cold    ☐ Foggy     ☐ Windy

## Drugs / Medications

| Qty | | Description | Strength |
|---|---|---|---|
| AM | PM | | |
| | | | |
| | | | |
| | | | |
| | | | |
| | | | |
| | | | |
| | | | |

## Vitamins / Herbs

| Qty | | Description | Strength |
|---|---|---|---|
| AM | PM | | |
| | | | |
| | | | |
| | | | |
| | | | |
| | | | |
| | | | |
| | | | |

MemoryMinder©

## Physical Activity

| Activity | Hours | Mins. |
|---|---|---|
| | | |
| | | |
| | | |

## Pain / Discomfort / Skin Changes

### Scale

1 Mild
2 Moderate
3 Severe
4 Very Severe
5 Worst Possible

Mark the area where the pain occurs with the number which corresponds to the intensity of the pain.

### In general, today I felt:

☐ Good
☐ Fair
☐ Poor

# Today's Conditions and Symptoms

Check the areas which apply and explain your conditions or symptoms in the space provided. See the *Symptoms Glossary* to help you describe your conditions.

☐ *Ears / Eyes / Nose*
_____

☐ *Mouth / Throat*
_____

☐ *Head / Neck / Back*
_____

☐ *Shoulders / Arms / Hands*
_____

☐ *Chest / Heart*
_____

☐ *Respiratory System*
_____

☐ *Digestive System*
_____

☐ *Hips / Legs / Feet*
_____

☐ *Male / Female Organs*
_____

☐ *Skin*
_____

☐ *Mood*
_____

☐ *Other*
_____
_____

## Comments
_____
_____
_____
_____

## Today's Diet

In columns A&B, list the nutritional facts you wish to monitor (i.e. fat, calories, sodium, sugar, protein, etc.)

☐ **Breakfast**

| | A | B |
|---|---|---|
| | | |
| | | |
| | | |
| | | |
| | | |
| Breakfast Totals | | |

☐ **Lunch**

| | A | B |
|---|---|---|
| | | |
| | | |
| | | |
| | | |
| | | |
| Lunch Totals | | |

☐ **Dinner**

| | A | B |
|---|---|---|
| | | |
| | | |
| | | |
| | | |
| | | |
| Dinner Totals | | |

☐ **Snacks**

| | A | B |
|---|---|---|
| | | |
| | | |
| | | |
| Snack Totals | | |

GRAND TOTALS FOR TODAY:

| A | B |
|---|---|
| | |

MemoryMinder©

|  | | Date |  | Day |
|---|---|---|---|---|

|  | AM | PM |
|---|---|---|
| Weight | | |
| Temperature | | |
| Blood Pressure | | |
| Sugar Level | | |
| Hours slept last night | Number of hours: | Sound ☐ Restless ☐ |
| Naps taken today | How many? | Total hours: |

## Today's Weather

☐ Hot　　☐ Sunny　　☐ Damp
☐ Warm　☐ Cloudy　☐ Rainy
☐ Cool　　☐ Overcast　☐ Snowy
☐ Cold　　☐ Foggy　　☐ Windy

## Drugs / Medications

| Qty | | Description | Strength |
|---|---|---|---|
| AM | PM | | |
| | | | |
| | | | |
| | | | |
| | | | |
| | | | |
| | | | |

## Vitamins / Herbs

| Qty | | Description | Strength |
|---|---|---|---|
| AM | PM | | |
| | | | |
| | | | |
| | | | |
| | | | |
| | | | |
| | | | |

MemoryMinder©

## Physical Activity

| Activity | Hours | Mins. |
|---|---|---|
| | | |
| | | |
| | | |

## Pain / Discomfort / Skin Changes

### Scale

1 Mild
2 Moderate
3 Severe
4 Very Severe
5 Worst Possible

Mark the area where the pain occurs with the number which corresponds to the intensity of the pain.

### In general, today I felt:

☐ Good
☐ Fair
☐ Poor

## Today's Conditions and Symptoms

Check the areas which apply and explain your conditions or symptoms in the space provided. See the *Symptoms Glossary* to help you describe your conditions.

☐ *Ears / Eyes / Nose*

_____

☐ *Mouth / Throat*

_____

☐ *Head / Neck / Back*

_____

☐ *Shoulders / Arms / Hands*

_____

☐ *Chest / Heart*

_____

☐ *Respiratory System*

_____

☐ *Digestive System*

_____

☐ *Hips / Legs / Feet*

_____

☐ *Male / Female Organs*

_____

☐ *Skin*

_____

☐ *Mood*

_____

☐ *Other*

_____
_____

## Comments

_____
_____
_____
_____

MemoryMinder©

## Today's Diet

In columns A&B, list the nutritional facts you wish to monitor (i.e. fat, calories, sodium, sugar, protein, etc.)

☐ **Breakfast**

| | A | B |
|---|---|---|
| | | |
| | | |
| | | |
| | | |
| | | |
| Breakfast Totals | | |

☐ **Lunch**

| | A | B |
|---|---|---|
| | | |
| | | |
| | | |
| | | |
| | | |
| Lunch Totals | | |

☐ **Dinner**

| | A | B |
|---|---|---|
| | | |
| | | |
| | | |
| | | |
| | | |
| Dinner Totals | | |

☐ **Snacks**

| | A | B |
|---|---|---|
| | | |
| | | |
| | | |
| Snack Totals | | |

GRAND TOTALS FOR TODAY:

| A | B |
|---|---|
| | |

| | | Date | | Day |
| --- | --- | --- | --- | --- |

## Today's Weather

- [ ] Hot
- [ ] Warm
- [ ] Cool
- [ ] Cold
- [ ] Sunny
- [ ] Cloudy
- [ ] Overcast
- [ ] Foggy
- [ ] Damp
- [ ] Rainy
- [ ] Snowy
- [ ] Windy

| | AM | PM |
| --- | --- | --- |
| Weight | | |
| Temperature | | |
| Blood Pressure | | |
| Sugar Level | | |
| Hours slept last night | Number of hours: | Sound [ ] Restless [ ] |
| Naps taken today | How many? | Total hours: |

## Drugs / Medications

| Qty | | Description | Strength |
| --- | --- | --- | --- |
| AM | PM | | |
| | | | |
| | | | |
| | | | |
| | | | |
| | | | |
| | | | |

## Vitamins / Herbs

| Qty | | Description | Strength |
| --- | --- | --- | --- |
| AM | PM | | |
| | | | |
| | | | |
| | | | |
| | | | |
| | | | |
| | | | |

MemoryMinder©

## Physical Activity

| Activity | Hours | Mins. |
| --- | --- | --- |
| | | |
| | | |
| | | |
| | | |

## Pain / Discomfort / Skin Changes

### Scale

1 Mild
2 Moderate
3 Severe
4 Very Severe
5 Worst Possible

Mark the area where the pain occurs with the number which corresponds to the intensity of the pain.

### In general, today I felt:

- [ ] Good
- [ ] Fair
- [ ] Poor

# Today's Conditions and Symptoms

Check the areas which apply and explain your conditions + symptoms in the space provided. See the *Symptoms Glossary* to help you describe your conditions.

☐ *Ears / Eyes / Nose*
_____

☐ *Mouth / Throat*
_____

☐ *Head / Neck / Back*
_____

☐ *Shoulders / Arms / Hands*
_____

☐ *Chest / Heart*
_____

☐ *Respiratory System*
_____

☐ *Digestive System*
_____

☐ *Hips / Legs / Feet*
_____

☐ *Male / Female Organs*
_____

☐ *Skin*
_____

☐ *Mood*
_____

☐ *Other*
_____
_____

## Comments
_____
_____
_____
_____

## Today's Diet

In columns A&B, list the nutritional facts you wish to monitor (i.e. fat, calories, sodium, sugar, protein, etc.)

| ☐ **Breakfast** | A | B |
|---|---|---|
| | | |
| | | |
| | | |
| | | |
| | | |
| Breakfast Totals | | |

| ☐ **Lunch** | | |
|---|---|---|
| | | |
| | | |
| | | |
| | | |
| | | |
| Lunch Totals | | |

| ☐ **Dinner** | | |
|---|---|---|
| | | |
| | | |
| | | |
| | | |
| | | |
| Dinner Totals | | |

| ☐ **Snacks** | | |
|---|---|---|
| | | |
| | | |
| | | |
| Snack Totals | | |

GRAND TOTALS FOR TODAY:

| A | B |
|---|---|
| | |

MemoryMinder©

| | Date | | Day |
|---|---|---|---|

## Today's Weather

- [ ] Hot
- [ ] Warm
- [ ] Cool
- [ ] Cold
- [ ] Sunny
- [ ] Cloudy
- [ ] Overcast
- [ ] Foggy
- [ ] Damp
- [ ] Rainy
- [ ] Snowy
- [ ] Windy

| | AM | PM |
|---|---|---|
| Weight | | |
| Temperature | | |
| Blood Pressure | | |
| Sugar Level | | |
| Hours slept last night | Number of hours: | Sound ☐ Restless ☐ |
| Naps taken today | How many? | Total hours: |

## Drugs / Medications

| Qty | | Description | Strength |
|---|---|---|---|
| AM | PM | | |
| | | | |
| | | | |
| | | | |
| | | | |
| | | | |
| | | | |
| | | | |

## Vitamins / Herbs

| Qty | | Description | Strength |
|---|---|---|---|
| AM | PM | | |
| | | | |
| | | | |
| | | | |
| | | | |
| | | | |
| | | | |
| | | | |

MemoryMinder©

## Physical Activity

| Activity | Hours | Mins. |
|---|---|---|
| | | |
| | | |
| | | |
| | | |

## Pain / Discomfort / Skin Changes

### Scale

1 Mild
2 Moderate
3 Severe
4 Very Severe
5 Worst Possible

Mark the area where the pain occurs with the number which corresponds to the intensity of the pain.

### In general, today I felt:

- [ ] Good
- [ ] Fair
- [ ] Poor

## Today's Conditions and Symptoms

Check the areas which apply and explain your conditions or symptoms in the space provided. See the *Symptoms Glossary* to help you describe your conditions.

☐ *Ears / Eyes / Nose*
_____
_____

☐ *Mouth / Throat*
_____
_____

☐ *Head / Neck / Back*
_____
_____

☐ *Shoulders / Arms / Hands*
_____
_____

☐ *Chest / Heart*
_____
_____

☐ *Respiratory System*
_____
_____

☐ *Digestive System*
_____
_____

☐ *Hips / Legs / Feet*
_____
_____

☐ *Male / Female Organs*
_____
_____

☐ *Skin*
_____
_____

☐ *Mood*
_____
_____

☐ *Other*
_____
_____
_____

## Comments
_____
_____
_____
_____

## Today's Diet

In columns A&B, list the nutritional facts you wish to monitor (i.e. fat, calories, sodium, sugar, protein, etc.)

| ☐ **Breakfast** | A | B |
|---|---|---|
| | | |
| | | |
| | | |
| | | |
| | | |
| Breakfast Totals | | |

| ☐ **Lunch** | | |
|---|---|---|
| | | |
| | | |
| | | |
| | | |
| | | |
| Lunch Totals | | |

| ☐ **Dinner** | | |
|---|---|---|
| | | |
| | | |
| | | |
| | | |
| | | |
| Dinner Totals | | |

| ☐ **Snacks** | | |
|---|---|---|
| | | |
| | | |
| | | |
| Snack Totals | | |

GRAND TOTALS FOR TODAY:

| A | B |
|---|---|
| | |

MemoryMinder©

_____ _____
Date                    Day

| | AM | PM |
|---|---|---|
| Weight | | |
| Temperature | | |
| Blood Pressure | | |
| Sugar Level | | |

## Today's Weather

- [ ] Hot
- [ ] Warm
- [ ] Cool
- [ ] Cold
- [ ] Sunny
- [ ] Cloudy
- [ ] Overcast
- [ ] Foggy
- [ ] Damp
- [ ] Rainy
- [ ] Snowy
- [ ] Windy

| Hours slept last night | Number of hours: | Sound [ ] Restless [ ] |
|---|---|---|
| Naps taken today | How many? | Total hours: |

## Drugs / Medications

| Qty | | Description | Strength |
|---|---|---|---|
| AM | PM | | |
| | | | |
| | | | |
| | | | |
| | | | |
| | | | |
| | | | |
| | | | |

## Vitamins / Herbs

| Qty | | Description | Strengt |
|---|---|---|---|
| AM | PM | | |
| | | | |
| | | | |
| | | | |
| | | | |
| | | | |
| | | | |
| | | | |

MemoryMinder©

## Physical Activity

| Activity | Hours | Mins |
|---|---|---|
| | | |
| | | |
| | | |
| | | |

## Pain / Discomfort / Skin Changes

### Scale

1 Mild
2 Moderate
3 Severe
4 Very Severe
5 Worst Possible

Mark the area where the pain occurs with the number which corresponds to the intensity of the pain.

### In general, today I felt:

- [ ] Good
- [ ] Fair
- [ ] Poor

## Today's Conditions and Symptoms

Check the areas which apply and explain your conditions or symptoms in the space provided. See the *Symptoms Glossary* to help you describe your conditions.

☐ *Ears / Eyes / Nose*

_____

☐ *Mouth / Throat*

_____

☐ *Head / Neck / Back*

_____

☐ *Shoulders / Arms / Hands*

_____

☐ *Chest / Heart*

_____

☐ *Respiratory System*

_____

☐ *Digestive System*

_____

☐ *Hips / Legs / Feet*

_____

☐ *Male / Female Organs*

_____

☐ *Skin*

_____

☐ *Mood*

_____

☐ *Other*

_____
_____

## Comments

_____
_____
_____
_____

## Today's Diet

In columns A&B, list the nutritional facts you wish to monitor (i.e. fat, calories, sodium, sugar, protein, etc.)

| ☐ *Breakfast* | A | B |
|---|---|---|
| | | |
| | | |
| | | |
| | | |
| | | |
| Breakfast Totals | | |

| ☐ *Lunch* | | |
|---|---|---|
| | | |
| | | |
| | | |
| | | |
| | | |
| Lunch Totals | | |

| ☐ *Dinner* | | |
|---|---|---|
| | | |
| | | |
| | | |
| | | |
| | | |
| Dinner Totals | | |

| ☐ *Snacks* | | |
|---|---|---|
| | | |
| | | |
| | | |
| Snack Totals | | |

GRAND TOTALS FOR TODAY:

| A | B |
|---|---|
| | |

MemoryMinder©

| | _____ | _____ |
|---|---|---|
| | Date | Day |

|  | AM | PM |
|---|---|---|
| Weight | | |
| Temperature | | |
| Blood Pressure | | |
| Sugar Level | | |
| Hours slept last night | Number of hours: | Sound ☐ Restless ☐ |
| Naps taken today | How many? | Total hours: |

## *Today's Weather*

☐ Hot  ☐ Sunny  ☐ Damp
☐ Warm  ☐ Cloudy  ☐ Rainy
☐ Cool  ☐ Overcast  ☐ Snowy
☐ Cold  ☐ Foggy  ☐ Windy

## *Drugs / Medications*

| Qty | | Description | Strength |
|---|---|---|---|
| AM | PM | | |
| | | | |
| | | | |
| | | | |
| | | | |
| | | | |
| | | | |
| | | | |

## *Vitamins / Herbs*

| Qty | | Description | Strength |
|---|---|---|---|
| AM | PM | | |
| | | | |
| | | | |
| | | | |
| | | | |
| | | | |
| | | | |

MemoryMinder©

## *Physical Activity*

| Activity | Hours | Mins |
|---|---|---|
| | | |
| | | |
| | | |

## *Pain / Discomfort / Skin Changes*

### Scale

1 Mild
2 Moderate
3 Severe
4 Very Severe
5 Worst Possible

Mark the area where the pain occurs with the number which corresponds to the intensity of the pain.

## *In general, today I felt:*

☐ Good
☐ Fair
☐ Poor

## Today's Conditions and Symptoms

Check the areas which apply and explain your conditions & symptoms in the space provided. See the *Symptoms Glossary* to help you describe your conditions.

☐ *Ears / Eyes / Nose*

☐ *Mouth / Throat*

☐ *Head / Neck / Back*

☐ *Shoulders / Arms / Hands*

☐ *Chest / Heart*

☐ *Respiratory System*

☐ *Digestive System*

☐ *Hips / Legs / Feet*

☐ *Male / Female Organs*

☐ *Skin*

☐ *Mood*

☐ *Other*

## Comments

## Today's Diet

In columns A&B, list the nutritional facts you wish to monitor (i.e. fat, calories, sodium, sugar, protein, etc.)

| ☐ *Breakfast* | A | B |
|---|---|---|
| | | |
| | | |
| | | |
| | | |
| | | |
| Breakfast Totals | | |

| ☐ *Lunch* | | |
|---|---|---|
| | | |
| | | |
| | | |
| | | |
| | | |
| Lunch Totals | | |

| ☐ *Dinner* | | |
|---|---|---|
| | | |
| | | |
| | | |
| | | |
| | | |
| Dinner Totals | | |

| ☐ *Snacks* | | |
|---|---|---|
| | | |
| | | |
| | | |
| Snack Totals | | |

GRAND TOTALS FOR TODAY:

| A | B |
|---|---|
| | |

MemoryMinder©

_____  _____
Date            Day

|  | AM | PM |
|---|---|---|
| Weight | | |
| Temperature | | |
| Blood Pressure | | |
| Sugar Level | | |
| Hours slept last night | Number of hours: | Sound ☐ Restless ☐ |
| Naps taken today | How many? | Total hours: |

## Today's Weather

☐ Hot      ☐ Sunny      ☐ Damp
☐ Warm     ☐ Cloudy     ☐ Rainy
☐ Cool     ☐ Overcast   ☐ Snowy
☐ Cold     ☐ Foggy      ☐ Windy

## Drugs / Medications

| Qty | | Description | Strength |
|---|---|---|---|
| AM | PM | | |
| | | | |
| | | | |
| | | | |
| | | | |
| | | | |
| | | | |
| | | | |

## Vitamins / Herbs

| Qty | | Description | Strength |
|---|---|---|---|
| AM | PM | | |
| | | | |
| | | | |
| | | | |
| | | | |
| | | | |
| | | | |
| | | | |

MemoryMinder©

## Physical Activity

| Activity | Hours | Mins. |
|---|---|---|
| | | |
| | | |
| | | |

## Pain / Discomfort / Skin Changes

### Scale

1 Mild
2 Moderate
3 Severe
4 Very Severe
5 Worst Possible

Mark the area where the pain occurs with the number which corresponds to the intensity of the pain.

### In general, today I felt:

☐ Good
☐ Fair
☐ Poor

## Today's Conditions and Symptoms

Check the areas which apply and explain your conditions or symptoms in the space provided. See the *Symptoms Glossary* to help you describe your conditions.

☐ *Ears / Eyes / Nose*
_____

☐ *Mouth / Throat*
_____

☐ *Head / Neck / Back*
_____

☐ *Shoulders / Arms / Hands*
_____

☐ *Chest / Heart*
_____

☐ *Respiratory System*
_____

☐ *Digestive System*
_____

☐ *Hips / Legs / Feet*
_____

☐ *Male / Female Organs*
_____

☐ *Skin*
_____

☐ *Mood*
_____

☐ *Other*
_____
_____

## Comments
_____
_____
_____
_____

## Today's Diet

In columns A&B, list the nutritional facts you wish to monitor (i.e. fat, calories, sodium, sugar, protein, etc.)

| ☐ **Breakfast** | A | B |
|---|---|---|
| | | |
| | | |
| | | |
| | | |
| | | |
| Breakfast Totals | | |

| ☐ **Lunch** | | |
|---|---|---|
| | | |
| | | |
| | | |
| | | |
| | | |
| Lunch Totals | | |

| ☐ **Dinner** | | |
|---|---|---|
| | | |
| | | |
| | | |
| | | |
| | | |
| Dinner Totals | | |

| ☐ **Snacks** | | |
|---|---|---|
| | | |
| | | |
| | | |
| Snack Totals | | |

GRAND TOTALS FOR TODAY:

| A | B |
|---|---|
| | |

Memory Minder©

| | AM | PM |
|---|---|---|
| Date _____ Day _____ | | |

## Today's Weather

- [ ] Hot
- [ ] Warm
- [ ] Cool
- [ ] Cold
- [ ] Sunny
- [ ] Cloudy
- [ ] Overcast
- [ ] Foggy
- [ ] Damp
- [ ] Rainy
- [ ] Snowy
- [ ] Windy

| | AM | PM |
|---|---|---|
| Weight | | |
| Temperature | | |
| Blood Pressure | | |
| Sugar Level | | |
| Hours slept last night | Number of hours: | Sound [ ] Restless [ ] |
| Naps taken today | How many? | Total hours: |

## Drugs / Medications

| Qty | | Description | Strength |
|---|---|---|---|
| AM | PM | | |
| | | | |
| | | | |
| | | | |
| | | | |
| | | | |
| | | | |
| | | | |

## Vitamins / Herbs

| Qty | | Description | Strength |
|---|---|---|---|
| AM | PM | | |
| | | | |
| | | | |
| | | | |
| | | | |
| | | | |
| | | | |
| | | | |

MemoryMinder©

## Physical Activity

| Activity | Hours | Mins. |
|---|---|---|
| | | |
| | | |
| | | |
| | | |

## Pain / Discomfort / Skin Changes

### Scale

1 Mild
2 Moderate
3 Severe
4 Very Severe
5 Worst Possible

Mark the area where the pain occurs with the number which corresponds to the intensity of the pain.

### In general, today I felt:

- [ ] Good
- [ ] Fair
- [ ] Poor

# Today's Conditions and Symptoms

Check the areas which apply and explain your conditions or symptoms in the space provided. See the *Symptoms Glossary* to help you describe your conditions.

☐ *Ears / Eyes / Nose*

_____

☐ *Mouth / Throat*

_____

☐ *Head / Neck / Back*

_____

☐ *Shoulders / Arms / Hands*

_____

☐ *Chest / Heart*

_____

☐ *Respiratory System*

_____

☐ *Digestive System*

_____

☐ *Hips / Legs / Feet*

_____

☐ *Male / Female Organs*

_____

☐ *Skin*

_____

☐ *Mood*

_____

☐ *Other*

_____
_____

# Comments

_____
_____
_____
_____

# Today's Diet

In columns A&B, list the nutritional facts you wish to monitor (i.e. fat, calories, sodium, sugar, protein, etc.)

| ☐ **Breakfast** | A | B |
|---|---|---|
| | | |
| | | |
| | | |
| | | |
| | | |
| Breakfast Totals | | |

| ☐ **Lunch** | | |
|---|---|---|
| | | |
| | | |
| | | |
| | | |
| | | |
| Lunch Totals | | |

| ☐ **Dinner** | | |
|---|---|---|
| | | |
| | | |
| | | |
| | | |
| | | |
| Dinner Totals | | |

| ☐ **Snacks** | | |
|---|---|---|
| | | |
| | | |
| | | |
| Snack Totals | | |

GRAND TOTALS FOR TODAY:

| A | B |
|---|---|
| | |

MemoryMinder©

_____ _____
Date                          Day

| | AM | PM |
|---|---|---|
| Weight | | |
| Temperature | | |
| Blood Pressure | | |
| Sugar Level | | |
| Hours slept last night | Number of hours: | Sound ☐ Restless ☐ |
| Naps taken today | How many? | Total hours: |

## Today's Weather

☐ Hot     ☐ Sunny      ☐ Damp
☐ Warm    ☐ Cloudy     ☐ Rainy
☐ Cool    ☐ Overcast   ☐ Snowy
☐ Cold    ☐ Foggy      ☐ Windy

## Drugs / Medications

| Qty | | Description | Strength |
|---|---|---|---|
| AM | PM | | |
| | | | |
| | | | |
| | | | |
| | | | |
| | | | |
| | | | |
| | | | |

## Vitamins / Herbs

| Qty | | Description | Strength |
|---|---|---|---|
| AM | PM | | |
| | | | |
| | | | |
| | | | |
| | | | |
| | | | |
| | | | |
| | | | |

MemoryMinder©

## Physical Activity

| Activity | Hours | Mins. |
|---|---|---|
| | | |
| | | |
| | | |

## Pain / Discomfort / Skin Changes

### Scale

1 Mild
2 Moderate
3 Severe
4 Very Severe
5 Worst Possible

Mark the area where the pain occurs with the number which corresponds to the intensity of the pain.

### In general, today I felt:

☐ Good
☐ Fair
☐ Poor

# Today's Conditions and Symptoms

Check the areas which apply and explain your conditions
or symptoms in the space provided. See the *Symptoms
Glossary* to help you describe your conditions.

☐ *Ears / Eyes / Nose*
_____

☐ *Mouth / Throat*
_____

☐ *Head / Neck / Back*
_____

☐ *Shoulders / Arms / Hands*
_____

☐ *Chest / Heart*
_____

☐ *Respiratory System*
_____

☐ *Digestive System*
_____

☐ *Hips / Legs / Feet*
_____

☐ *Male / Female Organs*
_____

☐ *Skin*
_____

☐ *Mood*
_____

☐ *Other*
_____
_____

## Comments
_____
_____
_____
_____

# Today's Diet

In columns A&B, list the nutritional
facts you wish to monitor (i.e. fat,
calories, sodium, sugar, protein, etc.)

| ☐ *Breakfast* | A | B |
|---|---|---|
| | | |
| | | |
| | | |
| | | |
| | | |
| Breakfast Totals | | |

| ☐ *Lunch* | | |
|---|---|---|
| | | |
| | | |
| | | |
| | | |
| | | |
| Lunch Totals | | |

| ☐ *Dinner* | | |
|---|---|---|
| | | |
| | | |
| | | |
| | | |
| | | |
| Dinner Totals | | |

| ☐ *Snacks* | | |
|---|---|---|
| | | |
| | | |
| | | |
| Snack Totals | | |

GRAND TOTALS FOR TODAY:

| A | B |
|---|---|
| | |

MemoryMinder©

_____  _____
       Date              Day

|               | AM | PM |
|---------------|----|----|
| Weight        |    |    |
| Temperature   |    |    |
| Blood Pressure |  /  |  /  |
| Sugar Level   |    |    |
| Hours slept last night | Number of hours: | Sound ☐ Restless ☐ |
| Naps taken today | How many? | Total hours: |

## Today's Weather

☐ Hot      ☐ Sunny     ☐ Damp
☐ Warm     ☐ Cloudy    ☐ Rainy
☐ Cool     ☐ Overcast  ☐ Snowy
☐ Cold     ☐ Foggy     ☐ Windy

## Drugs / Medications

| Qty | | Description | Strength |
|-----|-----|-------------|----------|
| AM | PM | | |
| | | | |
| | | | |
| | | | |
| | | | |
| | | | |
| | | | |

## Vitamins / Herbs

| Qty | | Description | Strength |
|-----|-----|-------------|----------|
| AM | PM | | |
| | | | |
| | | | |
| | | | |
| | | | |
| | | | |
| | | | |

MemoryMinder©

## Physical Activity

| Activity | Hours | Mins. |
|----------|-------|-------|
| | | |
| | | |
| | | |

## Pain / Discomfort / Skin Changes

### Scale

1 Mild
2 Moderate
3 Severe
4 Very Severe
5 Worst Possible

Mark the area where the pain occurs with the number which corresponds to the intensity of the pain.

## In general, today I felt:

☐ Good
☐ Fair
☐ Poor

## Today's Conditions and Symptoms

Check the areas which apply and explain your conditions or symptoms in the space provided. See the *Symptoms Glossary* to help you describe your conditions.

☐ *Ears / Eyes / Nose*
_____
_____

☐ *Mouth / Throat*
_____
_____

☐ *Head / Neck / Back*
_____
_____

☐ *Shoulders / Arms / Hands*
_____
_____

☐ *Chest / Heart*
_____
_____

☐ *Respiratory System*
_____
_____

☐ *Digestive System*
_____
_____

☐ *Hips / Legs / Feet*
_____
_____

☐ *Male / Female Organs*
_____
_____

☐ *Skin*
_____
_____

☐ *Mood*
_____
_____

☐ *Other*
_____
_____
_____

## Comments
_____
_____
_____
_____

## Today's Diet

In columns A&B, list the nutritional facts you wish to monitor (i.e. fat, calories, sodium, sugar, protein, etc.)

| ☐ *Breakfast* | A | B |
|---|---|---|
| | | |
| | | |
| | | |
| | | |
| | | |
| Breakfast Totals | | |

| ☐ *Lunch* | | |
|---|---|---|
| | | |
| | | |
| | | |
| | | |
| | | |
| Lunch Totals | | |

| ☐ *Dinner* | | |
|---|---|---|
| | | |
| | | |
| | | |
| | | |
| | | |
| Dinner Totals | | |

| ☐ *Snacks* | | |
|---|---|---|
| | | |
| | | |
| | | |
| Snack Totals | | |

GRAND TOTALS FOR TODAY:

| A | B |
|---|---|
| | |

MemoryMinder©

| | | AM | PM |
|---|---|---|---|
| Weight | | | |
| Temperature | | | |
| Blood Pressure | | | |
| Sugar Level | | | |
| Hours slept last night | Number of hours: | | Sound ☐ Restless ☐ |
| Naps taken today | How many? | | Total hours: |

_____  _____
Date                     Day

## Today's Weather

☐ Hot     ☐ Sunny     ☐ Damp
☐ Warm    ☐ Cloudy    ☐ Rainy
☐ Cool    ☐ Overcast  ☐ Snowy
☐ Cold    ☐ Foggy     ☐ Windy

## Drugs / Medications

| Qty | | Description | Strength |
|---|---|---|---|
| AM | PM | | |
| | | | |
| | | | |
| | | | |
| | | | |
| | | | |
| | | | |

## Vitamins / Herbs

| Qty | | Description | Strength |
|---|---|---|---|
| AM | PM | | |
| | | | |
| | | | |
| | | | |
| | | | |
| | | | |
| | | | |

MemoryMinder©

## Physical Activity

| Activity | Hours | Mins. |
|---|---|---|
| | | |
| | | |
| | | |
| | | |

## Pain / Discomfort / Skin Changes

### Scale

1 Mild
2 Moderate
3 Severe
4 Very Severe
5 Worst Possible

Mark the area where the pain occurs with the number which corresponds to the intensity of the pain.

### In general, today I felt:

☐ Good
☐ Fair
☐ Poor

## Today's Conditions and Symptoms

Check the areas which apply and explain your conditions or symptoms in the space provided. See the *Symptoms Glossary* to help you describe your conditions.

☐ *Ears / Eyes / Nose*
_____
_____

☐ *Mouth / Throat*
_____
_____

☐ *Head / Neck / Back*
_____
_____

☐ *Shoulders / Arms / Hands*
_____
_____

☐ *Chest / Heart*
_____
_____

☐ *Respiratory System*
_____
_____

☐ *Digestive System*
_____
_____

☐ *Hips / Legs / Feet*
_____
_____

☐ *Male / Female Organs*
_____
_____

☐ *Skin*
_____
_____

☐ *Mood*
_____
_____

☐ *Other*
_____
_____
_____

## Comments
_____
_____
_____
_____
_____

## Today's Diet

In columns A&B, list the nutritional facts you wish to monitor (i.e. fat, calories, sodium, sugar, protein, etc.)

| ☐ *Breakfast* | A | B |
|---|---|---|
|  |  |  |
|  |  |  |
|  |  |  |
|  |  |  |
|  |  |  |
| Breakfast Totals |  |  |

| ☐ *Lunch* | | |
|---|---|---|
|  |  |  |
|  |  |  |
|  |  |  |
|  |  |  |
|  |  |  |
| Lunch Totals |  |  |

| ☐ *Dinner* | | |
|---|---|---|
|  |  |  |
|  |  |  |
|  |  |  |
|  |  |  |
|  |  |  |
| Dinner Totals |  |  |

| ☐ *Snacks* | | |
|---|---|---|
|  |  |  |
|  |  |  |
|  |  |  |
| Snack Totals |  |  |

GRAND TOTALS FOR TODAY:

| A | B |
|---|---|
|  |  |

MemoryMinder©

_____ _____
Date          Day

|  | AM | PM |
|---|---|---|
| Weight | | |
| Temperature | | |
| Blood Pressure | | |
| Sugar Level | | |
| Hours slept last night | Number of hours: | Sound ☐ Restless ☐ |
| Naps taken today | How many? | Total hours: |

## Today's Weather

☐ Hot      ☐ Sunny     ☐ Damp
☐ Warm     ☐ Cloudy    ☐ Rainy
☐ Cool     ☐ Overcast  ☐ Snowy
☐ Cold     ☐ Foggy     ☐ Windy

## Drugs / Medications

| Qty | | Description | Strength |
|---|---|---|---|
| AM | PM | | |
| | | | |
| | | | |
| | | | |
| | | | |
| | | | |
| | | | |

## Vitamins / Herbs

| Qty | | Description | Strength |
|---|---|---|---|
| AM | PM | | |
| | | | |
| | | | |
| | | | |
| | | | |
| | | | |

MemoryMinder©

## Physical Activity

| Activity | Hours | Mins. |
|---|---|---|
| | | |
| | | |
| | | |
| | | |

## Pain / Discomfort / Skin Changes

### Scale
1 Mild
2 Moderate
3 Severe
4 Very Severe
5 Worst Possible

Mark the area where the pain occurs with the number which corresponds to the intensity of the pain.

### In general, today I felt:

☐ Good
☐ Fair
☐ Poor

## Today's Conditions and Symptoms

Check the areas which apply and explain your conditions or symptoms in the space provided. See the *Symptoms Glossary* to help you describe your conditions.

☐ *Ears / Eyes / Nose*
_____

☐ *Mouth / Throat*
_____

☐ *Head / Neck / Back*
_____

☐ *Shoulders / Arms / Hands*
_____

☐ *Chest / Heart*
_____

☐ *Respiratory System*
_____

☐ *Digestive System*
_____

☐ *Hips / Legs / Feet*
_____

☐ *Male / Female Organs*
_____

☐ *Skin*
_____

☐ *Mood*
_____

☐ *Other*
_____
_____

## Comments
_____
_____
_____
_____

## Today's Diet

In columns A&B, list the nutritional facts you wish to monitor (i.e. fat, calories, sodium, sugar, protein, etc.)

☐ *Breakfast*

| | A | B |
|---|---|---|
| | | |
| | | |
| | | |
| | | |
| | | |
| Breakfast Totals | | |

☐ *Lunch*

| | A | B |
|---|---|---|
| | | |
| | | |
| | | |
| | | |
| | | |
| Lunch Totals | | |

☐ *Dinner*

| | A | B |
|---|---|---|
| | | |
| | | |
| | | |
| | | |
| | | |
| Dinner Totals | | |

☐ *Snacks*

| | A | B |
|---|---|---|
| | | |
| | | |
| | | |
| Snack Totals | | |

GRAND TOTALS FOR TODAY:

| A | | B | |
|---|---|---|---|
| | | | |

MemoryMinder©

| | AM | PM |
|---|---|---|
| Weight | | |
| Temperature | | |
| Blood Pressure | | |
| Sugar Level | | |
| Hours slept last night | Number of hours: | Sound ☐ Restless ☐ |
| Naps taken today | How many? | Total hours: |

_____  _____
Date                    Day

## Today's Weather

☐ Hot      ☐ Sunny     ☐ Damp
☐ Warm     ☐ Cloudy    ☐ Rainy
☐ Cool     ☐ Overcast  ☐ Snowy
☐ Cold     ☐ Foggy     ☐ Windy

## Drugs / Medications

| Qty | | Description | Strength |
|---|---|---|---|
| AM | PM | | |
| | | | |
| | | | |
| | | | |
| | | | |
| | | | |
| | | | |

## Vitamins / Herbs

| Qty | | Description | Strengt |
|---|---|---|---|
| AM | PM | | |
| | | | |
| | | | |
| | | | |
| | | | |
| | | | |
| | | | |

MemoryMinder©

## Physical Activity

| Activity | Hours | Mins. |
|---|---|---|
| | | |
| | | |
| | | |

## Pain / Discomfort / Skin Changes

### Scale

1 Mild
2 Moderate
3 Severe
4 Very Severe
5 Worst Possible

Mark the area where the pain occurs with the number which corresponds to the intensity of the pain.

### In general, today I felt:

☐ Good
☐ Fair
☐ Poor

## Today's Conditions and Symptoms

Check the areas which apply and explain your conditions or symptoms in the space provided. See the *Symptoms Glossary* to help you describe your conditions.

☐ *Ears / Eyes / Nose*

_____

☐ *Mouth / Throat*

_____

☐ *Head / Neck / Back*

_____

☐ *Shoulders / Arms / Hands*

_____

☐ *Chest / Heart*

_____

☐ *Respiratory System*

_____

☐ *Digestive System*

_____

☐ *Hips / Legs / Feet*

_____

☐ *Male / Female Organs*

_____

☐ *Skin*

_____

☐ *Mood*

_____

☐ *Other*

_____

## Comments

_____
_____
_____
_____

MemoryMinder©

## Today's Diet

In columns A&B, list the nutritional facts you wish to monitor (i.e. fat, calories, sodium, sugar, protein, etc.)

☐ *Breakfast*    A    B

Breakfast Totals

☐ *Lunch*

Lunch Totals

☐ *Dinner*

Dinner Totals

☐ *Snacks*

Snack Totals

GRAND TOTALS FOR TODAY:

| A | B |
|---|---|
|   |   |

| | Date | | Day |
| --- | --- | --- | --- |

| | AM | PM |
| --- | --- | --- |
| Weight | | |
| Temperature | | |
| Blood Pressure | | |
| Sugar Level | | |
| Hours slept last night | Number of hours: | Sound ☐ Restless ☐ |
| Naps taken today | How many? | Total hours: |

## Today's Weather

☐ Hot   ☐ Sunny   ☐ Damp
☐ Warm   ☐ Cloudy   ☐ Rainy
☐ Cool   ☐ Overcast   ☐ Snowy
☐ Cold   ☐ Foggy   ☐ Windy

## Drugs / Medications

| Qty | | Description | Strength |
| --- | --- | --- | --- |
| AM | PM | | |
| | | | |
| | | | |
| | | | |
| | | | |
| | | | |
| | | | |
| | | | |

## Vitamins / Herbs

| Qty | | Description | Strengt |
| --- | --- | --- | --- |
| AM | PM | | |
| | | | |
| | | | |
| | | | |
| | | | |
| | | | |
| | | | |
| | | | |

MemoryMinder©

## Physical Activity

| Activity | Hours | Mins |
| --- | --- | --- |
| | | |
| | | |
| | | |

## Pain / Discomfort / Skin Changes

### Scale

1 Mild
2 Moderate
3 Severe
4 Very Severe
5 Worst Possible

Mark the area where the pain occurs with the number which corresponds to the intensity of the pain.

### In general, today I felt:

☐ Good
☐ Fair
☐ Poor

## Today's Conditions and Symptoms

Check the areas which apply and explain your conditions or symptoms in the space provided. See the *Symptoms Glossary* to help you describe your conditions.

☐ *Ears / Eyes / Nose*

_____

☐ *Mouth / Throat*

_____

☐ *Head / Neck / Back*

_____

☐ *Shoulders / Arms / Hands*

_____

☐ *Chest / Heart*

_____

☐ *Respiratory System*

_____

☐ *Digestive System*

_____

☐ *Hips / Legs / Feet*

_____

☐ *Male / Female Organs*

_____

☐ *Skin*

_____

☐ *Mood*

_____

☐ *Other*

_____

_____

## Comments

_____
_____
_____
_____
_____

MemoryMinder©

## Today's Diet

In columns A&B, list the nutritional facts you wish to monitor (i.e. fat, calories, sodium, sugar, protein, etc.)

☐ *Breakfast*

| | A | B |
|---|---|---|
| | | |
| | | |
| | | |
| | | |
| | | |
| Breakfast Totals | | |

☐ *Lunch*

| | A | B |
|---|---|---|
| | | |
| | | |
| | | |
| | | |
| | | |
| Lunch Totals | | |

☐ *Dinner*

| | A | B |
|---|---|---|
| | | |
| | | |
| | | |
| | | |
| | | |
| Dinner Totals | | |

☐ *Snacks*

| | A | B |
|---|---|---|
| | | |
| | | |
| | | |
| Snack Totals | | |

GRAND TOTALS FOR TODAY:

| A | B |
|---|---|
| | |

| | AM | PM |
|---|---|---|
| Weight | | |
| Temperature | | |
| Blood Pressure | | |
| Sugar Level | | |
| Hours slept last night | Number of hours: | Sound ☐ Restless ☐ |
| Naps taken today | How many? | Total hours: |

_____  _____
Date            Day

## Today's Weather

☐ Hot     ☐ Sunny     ☐ Damp
☐ Warm    ☐ Cloudy    ☐ Rainy
☐ Cool    ☐ Overcast  ☐ Snowy
☐ Cold    ☐ Foggy     ☐ Windy

## Drugs / Medications

| Qty | | Description | Strength |
|---|---|---|---|
| AM | PM | | |
| | | | |
| | | | |
| | | | |
| | | | |
| | | | |
| | | | |
| | | | |

## Vitamins / Herbs

| Qty | | Description | Strengt |
|---|---|---|---|
| AM | PM | | |
| | | | |
| | | | |
| | | | |
| | | | |
| | | | |
| | | | |

MemoryMinder©

## Physical Activity

| Activity | Hours | Mins. |
|---|---|---|
| | | |
| | | |
| | | |
| | | |

## Pain / Discomfort / Skin Changes

### Scale

1 Mild
2 Moderate
3 Severe
4 Very Severe
5 Worst Possible

Mark the area where the pain occurs with the number which corresponds to the intensity of the pain.

### In general, today I felt:

☐ Good
☐ Fair
☐ Poor

## Today's Conditions and Symptoms

Check the areas which apply and explain your conditions symptoms in the space provided. See the *Symptoms Glossary* to help you describe your conditions.

☐ *Ears / Eyes / Nose*

---

☐ *Mouth / Throat*

---

☐ *Head / Neck / Back*

---

☐ *Shoulders / Arms / Hands*

---

☐ *Chest / Heart*

---

☐ *Respiratory System*

---

☐ *Digestive System*

---

☐ *Hips / Legs / Feet*

---

☐ *Male / Female Organs*

---

☐ *Skin*

---

☐ *Mood*

---

☐ *Other*

---

## Comments

---

## Today's Diet

In columns A&B, list the nutritional facts you wish to monitor (i.e. fat, calories, sodium, sugar, protein, etc.)

| ☐ **Breakfast** | A | B |
|---|---|---|
| | | |
| | | |
| | | |
| | | |
| | | |
| Breakfast Totals | | |

| ☐ **Lunch** | | |
|---|---|---|
| | | |
| | | |
| | | |
| | | |
| | | |
| Lunch Totals | | |

| ☐ **Dinner** | | |
|---|---|---|
| | | |
| | | |
| | | |
| | | |
| | | |
| Dinner Totals | | |

| ☐ **Snacks** | | |
|---|---|---|
| | | |
| | | |
| | | |
| Snack Totals | | |

| GRAND TOTALS FOR TODAY: | |
|---|---|
| A | B |

MemoryMinder©

| | Date | | Day |
|---|---|---|---|

|  | AM | PM |
|---|---|---|
| Weight | | |
| Temperature | | |
| Blood Pressure | | |
| Sugar Level | | |
| Hours slept last night | Number of hours: | Sound ☐ Restless ☐ |
| Naps taken today | How many? | Total hours: |

## Today's Weather

☐ Hot   ☐ Sunny   ☐ Damp
☐ Warm   ☐ Cloudy   ☐ Rainy
☐ Cool   ☐ Overcast   ☐ Snowy
☐ Cold   ☐ Foggy   ☐ Windy

## Drugs / Medications

| Qty | | Description | Strength |
|---|---|---|---|
| AM | PM | | |
| | | | |
| | | | |
| | | | |
| | | | |
| | | | |
| | | | |
| | | | |

## Vitamins / Herbs

| Qty | | Description | Strength |
|---|---|---|---|
| AM | PM | | |
| | | | |
| | | | |
| | | | |
| | | | |
| | | | |
| | | | |

MemoryMinder©

## Physical Activity

| Activity | Hours | Mins. |
|---|---|---|
| | | |
| | | |
| | | |

## Pain / Discomfort / Skin Changes

### Scale

1 Mild
2 Moderate
3 Severe
4 Very Severe
5 Worst Possible

Mark the area where the pain occurs with the number which corresponds to the intensity of the pain.

### In general, today I felt:

☐ Good
☐ Fair
☐ Poor

## Today's Conditions and Symptoms

Check the areas which apply and explain your conditions or symptoms in the space provided. See the *Symptoms Glossary* to help you describe your conditions.

☐ *Ears / Eyes / Nose*

_____

☐ *Mouth / Throat*

_____

☐ *Head / Neck / Back*

_____

☐ *Shoulders / Arms / Hands*

_____

☐ *Chest / Heart*

_____

☐ *Respiratory System*

_____

☐ *Digestive System*

_____

☐ *Hips / Legs / Feet*

_____

☐ *Male / Female Organs*

_____

☐ *Skin*

_____

☐ *Mood*

_____

☐ *Other*

_____
_____

## Comments

_____
_____
_____
_____
_____

MemoryMinder©

## Today's Diet

In columns A&B, list the nutritional facts you wish to monitor (i.e. fat, calories, sodium, sugar, protein, etc.)

| ☐ **Breakfast** | A | B |
|---|---|---|
| | | |
| | | |
| | | |
| | | |
| | | |
| Breakfast Totals | | |

| ☐ **Lunch** | | |
|---|---|---|
| | | |
| | | |
| | | |
| | | |
| | | |
| Lunch Totals | | |

| ☐ **Dinner** | | |
|---|---|---|
| | | |
| | | |
| | | |
| | | |
| | | |
| Dinner Totals | | |

| ☐ **Snacks** | | |
|---|---|---|
| | | |
| | | |
| | | |
| Snack Totals | | |

GRAND TOTALS FOR TODAY:

| A | B |
|---|---|
| | |

| | Date | Day |
|---|---|---|

| | AM | PM |
|---|---|---|
| Weight | | |
| Temperature | | |
| Blood Pressure | | |
| Sugar Level | | |
| Hours slept last night | Number of hours: | Sound ☐ Restless ☐ |
| Naps taken today | How many? | Total hours: |

## Today's Weather

☐ Hot    ☐ Sunny    ☐ Damp
☐ Warm    ☐ Cloudy    ☐ Rainy
☐ Cool    ☐ Overcast    ☐ Snowy
☐ Cold    ☐ Foggy    ☐ Windy

## Drugs / Medications

| Qty | | Description | Strength |
|---|---|---|---|
| AM | PM | | |
| | | | |
| | | | |
| | | | |
| | | | |
| | | | |
| | | | |
| | | | |

## Vitamins / Herbs

| Qty | | Description | Strength |
|---|---|---|---|
| AM | PM | | |
| | | | |
| | | | |
| | | | |
| | | | |
| | | | |
| | | | |
| | | | |

MemoryMinder©

## Physical Activity

| Activity | Hours | Mins |
|---|---|---|
| | | |
| | | |
| | | |

## Pain / Discomfort / Skin Changes

### Scale

1 Mild
2 Moderate
3 Severe
4 Very Severe
5 Worst Possible

Mark the area where the pain occurs with the number which corresponds to the intensity of the pain.

### In general, today I felt:

☐ Good
☐ Fair
☐ Poor

# Today's Conditions and Symptoms

Check the areas which apply and explain your conditions or symptoms in the space provided. See the *Symptoms Glossary* to help you describe your conditions.

☐ **Ears / Eyes / Nose**

_____

☐ **Mouth / Throat**

_____

☐ **Head / Neck / Back**

_____

☐ **Shoulders / Arms / Hands**

_____

☐ **Chest / Heart**

_____

☐ **Respiratory System**

_____

☐ **Digestive System**

_____

☐ **Hips / Legs / Feet**

_____

☐ **Male / Female Organs**

_____

☐ **Skin**

_____

☐ **Mood**

_____

☐ **Other**

_____
_____

## Comments

_____
_____
_____
_____

MemoryMinder©

# Today's Diet

In columns A&B, list the nutritional facts you wish to monitor (i.e. fat, calories, sodium, sugar, protein, etc.)

☐ **Breakfast**     A     B

Breakfast Totals

☐ **Lunch**

Lunch Totals

☐ **Dinner**

Dinner Totals

☐ **Snacks**

Snack Totals

GRAND TOTALS FOR TODAY:

| A | B |
|---|---|
|   |   |

| | Date | | Day |
|---|---|---|---|

## Today's Weather

| | | | | | |
|---|---|---|---|---|---|
| ☐ | Hot | ☐ | Sunny | ☐ | Damp |
| ☐ | Warm | ☐ | Cloudy | ☐ | Rainy |
| ☐ | Cool | ☐ | Overcast | ☐ | Snowy |
| ☐ | Cold | ☐ | Foggy | ☐ | Windy |

| | AM | PM |
|---|---|---|
| Weight | | |
| Temperature | | |
| Blood Pressure | | |
| Sugar Level | | |
| Hours slept last night | Number of hours: | Sound ☐ Restless ☐ |
| Naps taken today | How many? | Total hours: |

## Drugs / Medications

| Qty | | Description | Strength |
|---|---|---|---|
| AM | PM | | |
| | | | |
| | | | |
| | | | |
| | | | |
| | | | |
| | | | |

## Vitamins / Herbs

| Qty | | Description | Strength |
|---|---|---|---|
| AM | PM | | |
| | | | |
| | | | |
| | | | |
| | | | |
| | | | |
| | | | |

MemoryMinder©

## Physical Activity

| Activity | Hours | Mins. |
|---|---|---|
| | | |
| | | |
| | | |
| | | |

## Pain / Discomfort / Skin Changes

### Scale

1 Mild
2 Moderate
3 Severe
4 Very Severe
5 Worst Possible

Mark the area where the pain occurs with the number which corresponds to the intensity of the pain.

### In general, today I felt:

☐ Good

☐ Fair

☐ Poor

## Today's Conditions and Symptoms

Check the areas which apply and explain your conditions or symptoms in the space provided. See the *Symptoms Glossary* to help you describe your conditions.

☐ *Ears / Eyes / Nose*
_____
_____

☐ *Mouth / Throat*
_____
_____

☐ *Head / Neck / Back*
_____
_____

☐ *Shoulders / Arms / Hands*
_____
_____

☐ *Chest / Heart*
_____
_____

☐ *Respiratory System*
_____
_____

☐ *Digestive System*
_____
_____

☐ *Hips / Legs / Feet*
_____
_____

☐ *Male / Female Organs*
_____
_____

☐ *Skin*
_____
_____

☐ *Mood*
_____
_____

☐ *Other*
_____
_____
_____

## Comments
_____
_____
_____
_____

MemoryMinder©

## Today's Diet

In columns A&B, list the nutritional facts you wish to monitor (i.e. fat, calories, sodium, sugar, protein, etc.)

| ☐ *Breakfast* | A | B |
|---|---|---|
| | | |
| | | |
| | | |
| | | |
| | | |
| Breakfast Totals | | |

| ☐ *Lunch* | | |
|---|---|---|
| | | |
| | | |
| | | |
| | | |
| | | |
| Lunch Totals | | |

| ☐ *Dinner* | | |
|---|---|---|
| | | |
| | | |
| | | |
| | | |
| | | |
| Dinner Totals | | |

| ☐ *Snacks* | | |
|---|---|---|
| | | |
| | | |
| | | |
| Snack Totals | | |

GRAND TOTALS FOR TODAY:

| A | B |
|---|---|
| | |

| | Date | | Day |
|---|---|---|---|

## Today's Weather

| | | |
|---|---|---|
| ☐ Hot | ☐ Sunny | ☐ Damp |
| ☐ Warm | ☐ Cloudy | ☐ Rainy |
| ☐ Cool | ☐ Overcast | ☐ Snowy |
| ☐ Cold | ☐ Foggy | ☐ Windy |

| | AM | PM |
|---|---|---|
| Weight | | |
| Temperature | | |
| Blood Pressure | | |
| Sugar Level | | |
| Hours slept last night | Number of hours: | Sound ☐ Restless ☐ |
| Naps taken today | How many? | Total hours: |

## Drugs / Medications

| Qty | | Description | Strength |
|---|---|---|---|
| AM | PM | | |
| | | | |
| | | | |
| | | | |
| | | | |
| | | | |
| | | | |

## Vitamins / Herbs

| Qty | | Description | Strength |
|---|---|---|---|
| AM | PM | | |
| | | | |
| | | | |
| | | | |
| | | | |
| | | | |
| | | | |

MemoryMinder©

## Physical Activity

| Activity | Hours | Mins. |
|---|---|---|
| | | |
| | | |
| | | |

## Pain / Discomfort / Skin Changes

### Scale

1 Mild
2 Moderate
3 Severe
4 Very Severe
5 Worst Possible

Mark the area where the pain occurs with the number which corresponds to the intensity of the pain.

### In general, today I felt:

☐ Good

☐ Fair

☐ Poor

## Today's Conditions and Symptoms

Check the areas which apply and explain your conditions or symptoms in the space provided. See the *Symptoms Glossary* to help you describe your conditions.

☐ *Ears / Eyes / Nose*

_____

☐ *Mouth / Throat*

_____

☐ *Head / Neck / Back*

_____

☐ *Shoulders / Arms / Hands*

_____

☐ *Chest / Heart*

_____

☐ *Respiratory System*

_____

☐ *Digestive System*

_____

☐ *Hips / Legs / Feet*

_____

☐ *Male / Female Organs*

_____

☐ *Skin*

_____

☐ *Mood*

_____

☐ *Other*

_____
_____

## Comments

_____
_____
_____
_____

MemoryMinder©

## Today's Diet

In columns A&B, list the nutritional facts you wish to monitor (i.e. fat, calories, sodium, sugar, protein, etc.)

☐ **Breakfast**

|  | A | B |
|---|---|---|
|  |  |  |
|  |  |  |
|  |  |  |
|  |  |  |
|  |  |  |
| Breakfast Totals |  |  |

☐ **Lunch**

|  | A | B |
|---|---|---|
|  |  |  |
|  |  |  |
|  |  |  |
|  |  |  |
|  |  |  |
| Lunch Totals |  |  |

☐ **Dinner**

|  | A | B |
|---|---|---|
|  |  |  |
|  |  |  |
|  |  |  |
|  |  |  |
|  |  |  |
| Dinner Totals |  |  |

☐ **Snacks**

|  | A | B |
|---|---|---|
|  |  |  |
|  |  |  |
|  |  |  |
| Snack Totals |  |  |

GRAND TOTALS FOR TODAY:

| A | B |
|---|---|
|  |  |

| | | Date | | | Day | |
|---|---|---|---|---|---|---|

## Today's Weather

- [ ] Hot
- [ ] Warm
- [ ] Cool
- [ ] Cold
- [ ] Sunny
- [ ] Cloudy
- [ ] Overcast
- [ ] Foggy
- [ ] Damp
- [ ] Rainy
- [ ] Snowy
- [ ] Windy

| | AM | PM |
|---|---|---|
| Weight | | |
| Temperature | | |
| Blood Pressure | | |
| Sugar Level | | |
| Hours slept last night | Number of hours: | Sound ☐ Restless ☐ |
| Naps taken today | How many? | Total hours: |

## Drugs / Medications

| Qty | | Description | Strength |
|---|---|---|---|
| AM | PM | | |
| | | | |
| | | | |
| | | | |
| | | | |
| | | | |
| | | | |
| | | | |

## Vitamins / Herbs

| Qty | | Description | Strengt |
|---|---|---|---|
| AM | PM | | |
| | | | |
| | | | |
| | | | |
| | | | |
| | | | |
| | | | |

MemoryMinder©

## Physical Activity

| Activity | Hours | Mins. |
|---|---|---|
| | | |
| | | |
| | | |
| | | |

## Pain / Discomfort / Skin Changes

### Scale

1 Mild
2 Moderate
3 Severe
4 Very Severe
5 Worst Possible

Mark the area where the pain occurs with the number which corresponds to the intensity of the pain.

### In general, today I felt:

- [ ] Good
- [ ] Fair
- [ ] Poor

## Today's Conditions and Symptoms

Check the areas which apply and explain your conditions symptoms in the space provided. See the *Symptoms Glossary* to help you describe your conditions.

☐ *Ears / Eyes / Nose*
_____
_____

☐ *Mouth / Throat*
_____
_____

☐ *Head / Neck / Back*
_____
_____

☐ *Shoulders / Arms / Hands*
_____
_____

☐ *Chest / Heart*
_____
_____

☐ *Respiratory System*
_____
_____

☐ *Digestive System*
_____
_____

☐ *Hips / Legs / Feet*
_____
_____

☐ *Male / Female Organs*
_____
_____

☐ *Skin*
_____
_____

☐ *Mood*
_____
_____

☐ *Other*
_____
_____
_____

## Comments
_____
_____
_____
_____

MemoryMinder©

## Today's Diet

In columns A&B, list the nutritional facts you wish to monitor (i.e. fat, calories, sodium, sugar, protein, etc.)

| ☐ *Breakfast* | A | B |
|---|---|---|
| | | |
| | | |
| | | |
| | | |
| | | |
| Breakfast Totals | | |

| ☐ *Lunch* | | |
|---|---|---|
| | | |
| | | |
| | | |
| | | |
| | | |
| Lunch Totals | | |

| ☐ *Dinner* | | |
|---|---|---|
| | | |
| | | |
| | | |
| | | |
| | | |
| Dinner Totals | | |

| ☐ *Snacks* | | |
|---|---|---|
| | | |
| | | |
| | | |
| Snack Totals | | |

GRAND TOTALS FOR TODAY:

| A | B |
|---|---|
| | |

| | | |
|---|---|---|
| _____ | _____ | |
| Date | Day | |

| | AM | PM |
|---|---|---|
| Weight | | |
| Temperature | | |
| Blood Pressure | | |
| Sugar Level | | |
| Hours slept last night | Number of hours: | Sound ☐ Restless ☐ |
| Naps taken today | How many? | Total hours: |

## Today's Weather

| | | |
|---|---|---|
| ☐ Hot | ☐ Sunny | ☐ Damp |
| ☐ Warm | ☐ Cloudy | ☐ Rainy |
| ☐ Cool | ☐ Overcast | ☐ Snowy |
| ☐ Cold | ☐ Foggy | ☐ Windy |

## Drugs / Medications

| Qty | | Description | Strength |
|---|---|---|---|
| AM | PM | | |
| | | | |
| | | | |
| | | | |
| | | | |
| | | | |
| | | | |

## Vitamins / Herbs

| Qty | | Description | Strengt |
|---|---|---|---|
| AM | PM | | |
| | | | |
| | | | |
| | | | |
| | | | |
| | | | |
| | | | |

MemoryMinder©

## Physical Activity

| Activity | Hours | Mins. |
|---|---|---|
| | | |
| | | |
| | | |
| | | |

## Pain / Discomfort / Skin Changes

### Scale

1 Mild
2 Moderate
3 Severe
4 Very Severe
5 Worst Possible

Mark the area where the pain occurs with the number which corresponds to the intensity of the pain.

### In general, today I felt:

☐ Good

☐ Fair

☐ Poor

## Today's Conditions and Symptoms

Check the areas which apply and explain your conditions or symptoms in the space provided. See the *Symptoms Glossary* to help you describe your conditions.

☐ *Ears / Eyes / Nose*

_____

☐ *Mouth / Throat*

_____

☐ *Head / Neck / Back*

_____

☐ *Shoulders / Arms / Hands*

_____

☐ *Chest / Heart*

_____

☐ *Respiratory System*

_____

☐ *Digestive System*

_____

☐ *Hips / Legs / Feet*

_____

☐ *Male / Female Organs*

_____

☐ *Skin*

_____

☐ *Mood*

_____

☐ *Other*

_____
_____

## Comments

_____
_____
_____
_____

MemoryMinder©

## Today's Diet

In columns A&B, list the nutritional facts you wish to monitor (i.e. fat, calories, sodium, sugar, protein, etc.)

☐ *Breakfast*     A     B

Breakfast Totals

☐ *Lunch*

Lunch Totals

☐ *Dinner*

Dinner Totals

☐ *Snacks*

Snack Totals

GRAND TOTALS FOR TODAY:

A _____     B _____

|  | | Date | | | Day |
| --- | --- | --- | --- | --- | --- |

|  | AM | PM |
| --- | --- | --- |
| Weight | | |
| Temperature | | |
| Blood Pressure | | |
| Sugar Level | | |
| Hours slept last night | Number of hours: | Sound ☐ Restless ☐ |
| Naps taken today | How many? | Total hours: |

## Today's Weather

| | | | | | |
| --- | --- | --- | --- | --- | --- |
| ☐ Hot | ☐ Sunny | ☐ Damp |
| ☐ Warm | ☐ Cloudy | ☐ Rainy |
| ☐ Cool | ☐ Overcast | ☐ Snowy |
| ☐ Cold | ☐ Foggy | ☐ Windy |

## Drugs / Medications

| Qty | | Description | Strength |
| --- | --- | --- | --- |
| AM | PM | | |
| | | | |
| | | | |
| | | | |
| | | | |
| | | | |
| | | | |
| | | | |

## Vitamins / Herbs

| Qty | | Description | Strengt |
| --- | --- | --- | --- |
| AM | PM | | |
| | | | |
| | | | |
| | | | |
| | | | |
| | | | |
| | | | |

MemoryMinder©

## Physical Activity

| Activity | Hours | Mins. |
| --- | --- | --- |
| | | |
| | | |
| | | |
| | | |

## Pain / Discomfort / Skin Changes

### Scale

1 Mild
2 Moderate
3 Severe
4 Very Severe
5 Worst Possible

Mark the area where the pain occurs with the number which corresponds to the intensity of the pain.

### In general, today I felt:

☐ Good

☐ Fair

☐ Poor

## Today's Conditions and Symptoms

Check the areas which apply and explain your conditions
& symptoms in the space provided. See the *Symptoms
Glossary* to help you describe your conditions.

☐ *Ears / Eyes / Nose*
_____

☐ *Mouth / Throat*
_____

☐ *Head / Neck / Back*
_____

☐ *Shoulders / Arms / Hands*
_____

☐ *Chest / Heart*
_____

☐ *Respiratory System*
_____

☐ *Digestive System*
_____

☐ *Hips / Legs / Feet*
_____

☐ *Male / Female Organs*
_____

☐ *Skin*
_____

☐ *Mood*
_____

☐ *Other*
_____
_____

## Comments
_____
_____
_____
_____

MemoryMinder©

## Today's Diet

In columns A&B, list the nutritional
facts you wish to monitor (i.e. fat,
calories, sodium, sugar, protein, etc.)

| ☐ *Breakfast* | A | B |
|---|---|---|
| | | |
| | | |
| | | |
| | | |
| | | |
| Breakfast Totals | | |

| ☐ *Lunch* | | |
|---|---|---|
| | | |
| | | |
| | | |
| | | |
| | | |
| Lunch Totals | | |

| ☐ *Dinner* | | |
|---|---|---|
| | | |
| | | |
| | | |
| | | |
| | | |
| Dinner Totals | | |

| ☐ *Snacks* | | |
|---|---|---|
| | | |
| | | |
| | | |
| Snack Totals | | |

GRAND TOTALS FOR TODAY:

| A | B |
|---|---|
| | |

| | AM | PM |
|---|---|---|
| Weight | | |
| Temperature | | |
| Blood Pressure | | |
| Sugar Level | | |
| Hours slept last night | Number of hours: | Sound ☐ Restless ☐ |
| Naps taken today | How many? | Total hours: |

_____  _____
Date              Day

## Today's Weather

- ☐ Hot
- ☐ Warm
- ☐ Cool
- ☐ Cold
- ☐ Sunny
- ☐ Cloudy
- ☐ Overcast
- ☐ Foggy
- ☐ Damp
- ☐ Rainy
- ☐ Snowy
- ☐ Windy

## Drugs / Medications

| Qty | | Description | Strength |
|---|---|---|---|
| AM | PM | | |
| | | | |
| | | | |
| | | | |
| | | | |
| | | | |
| | | | |
| | | | |

## Vitamins / Herbs

| Qty | | Description | Strength |
|---|---|---|---|
| AM | PM | | |
| | | | |
| | | | |
| | | | |
| | | | |
| | | | |
| | | | |
| | | | |

MemoryMinder©

## Physical Activity

| Activity | Hours | Mins. |
|---|---|---|
| | | |
| | | |
| | | |

## Pain / Discomfort / Skin Changes

### Scale

1 Mild
2 Moderate
3 Severe
4 Very Severe
5 Worst Possible

Mark the area where the pain occurs with the number which corresponds to the intensity of the pain.

### In general, today I felt:

- ☐ Good
- ☐ Fair
- ☐ Poor

## Today's Conditions and Symptoms

Check the areas which apply and explain your conditions or symptoms in the space provided. See the *Symptoms Glossary* to help you describe your conditions.

☐ *Ears / Eyes / Nose*
_____
_____

☐ *Mouth / Throat*
_____
_____

☐ *Head / Neck / Back*
_____
_____

☐ *Shoulders / Arms / Hands*
_____
_____

☐ *Chest / Heart*
_____
_____

☐ *Respiratory System*
_____
_____

☐ *Digestive System*
_____
_____

☐ *Hips / Legs / Feet*
_____
_____

☐ *Male / Female Organs*
_____
_____

☐ *Skin*
_____
_____

☐ *Mood*
_____
_____

☐ *Other*
_____
_____
_____

## Comments
_____
_____
_____
_____

## Today's Diet

In columns A&B, list the nutritional facts you wish to monitor (i.e. fat, calories, sodium, sugar, protein, etc.)

☐ **Breakfast**

|  | A | B |
|---|---|---|
|  |  |  |
|  |  |  |
|  |  |  |
|  |  |  |
| Breakfast Totals |  |  |

☐ **Lunch**

|  | A | B |
|---|---|---|
|  |  |  |
|  |  |  |
|  |  |  |
|  |  |  |
| Lunch Totals |  |  |

☐ **Dinner**

|  | A | B |
|---|---|---|
|  |  |  |
|  |  |  |
|  |  |  |
|  |  |  |
| Dinner Totals |  |  |

☐ **Snacks**

|  | A | B |
|---|---|---|
|  |  |  |
|  |  |  |
| Snack Totals |  |  |

GRAND TOTALS FOR TODAY:

| A | B |
|---|---|
|  |  |

MemoryMinder©

| | AM | PM |
|---|---|---|
| Weight | | |
| Temperature | | |
| Blood Pressure | | |
| Sugar Level | | |

_____ _____
Date                Day

## Today's Weather

- [ ] Hot
- [ ] Warm
- [ ] Cool
- [ ] Cold
- [ ] Sunny
- [ ] Cloudy
- [ ] Overcast
- [ ] Foggy
- [ ] Damp
- [ ] Rainy
- [ ] Snowy
- [ ] Windy

| Hours slept last night | Number of hours: | Sound / Restless |
| Naps taken today | How many? | Total hours: |

## Drugs / Medications

| Qty | | Description | Strength |
|---|---|---|---|
| AM | PM | | |
| | | | |
| | | | |
| | | | |
| | | | |
| | | | |
| | | | |

## Vitamins / Herbs

| Qty | | Description | Strength |
|---|---|---|---|
| AM | PM | | |
| | | | |
| | | | |
| | | | |
| | | | |
| | | | |
| | | | |

MemoryMinder©

## Physical Activity

| Activity | Hours | Mins. |
|---|---|---|
| | | |
| | | |
| | | |
| | | |

## Pain / Discomfort / Skin Changes

### Scale

1 Mild
2 Moderate
3 Severe
4 Very Severe
5 Worst Possible

Mark the area where the pain occurs with the number which corresponds to the intensity of the pain.

### In general, today I felt:

- [ ] Good
- [ ] Fair
- [ ] Poor

## Today's Conditions and Symptoms

Check the areas which apply and explain your conditions or symptoms in the space provided. See the *Symptoms Glossary* to help you describe your conditions.

◻ *Ears / Eyes / Nose*
_____
_____

◻ *Mouth / Throat*
_____
_____

◻ *Head / Neck / Back*
_____
_____

◻ *Shoulders / Arms / Hands*
_____
_____

◻ *Chest / Heart*
_____
_____

◻ *Respiratory System*
_____
_____

◻ *Digestive System*
_____
_____

◻ *Hips / Legs / Feet*
_____
_____

◻ *Male / Female Organs*
_____
_____

◻ *Skin*
_____
_____

◻ *Mood*
_____
_____

◻ *Other*
_____
_____
_____

## Comments
_____
_____
_____
_____

## Today's Diet

In columns A&B, list the nutritional facts you wish to monitor (i.e. fat, calories, sodium, sugar, protein, etc.)

| ◻ **Breakfast** | A | B |
|---|---|---|
|  |  |  |
|  |  |  |
|  |  |  |
|  |  |  |
|  |  |  |
| Breakfast Totals |  |  |

| ◻ **Lunch** |  |  |
|---|---|---|
|  |  |  |
|  |  |  |
|  |  |  |
|  |  |  |
|  |  |  |
| Lunch Totals |  |  |

| ◻ **Dinner** |  |  |
|---|---|---|
|  |  |  |
|  |  |  |
|  |  |  |
|  |  |  |
|  |  |  |
| Dinner Totals |  |  |

| ◻ **Snacks** |  |  |
|---|---|---|
|  |  |  |
|  |  |  |
|  |  |  |
| Snack Totals |  |  |

| GRAND TOTALS FOR TODAY: | |
|---|---|
| A | B |

MemoryMinder©

|        | Date | Day |
|--------|------|-----|

| | AM | PM |
|---|---|---|
| Weight | | |
| Temperature | | |
| Blood Pressure | | |
| Sugar Level | | |
| Hours slept last night | Number of hours: | Sound ☐ Restless ☐ |
| Naps taken today | How many? | Total hours: |

## Today's Weather

☐ Hot   ☐ Sunny    ☐ Damp
☐ Warm  ☐ Cloudy   ☐ Rainy
☐ Cool  ☐ Overcast ☐ Snowy
☐ Cold  ☐ Foggy    ☐ Windy

## Drugs / Medications

| Qty | | Description | Strength |
|-----|-----|-------------|----------|
| AM | PM | | |
| | | | |
| | | | |
| | | | |
| | | | |
| | | | |
| | | | |

## Vitamins / Herbs

| Qty | | Description | Strength |
|-----|-----|-------------|----------|
| AM | PM | | |
| | | | |
| | | | |
| | | | |
| | | | |
| | | | |
| | | | |

MemoryMinder©

## Physical Activity

| Activity | Hours | Mins. |
|----------|-------|-------|
| | | |
| | | |
| | | |

## Pain / Discomfort / Skin Changes

### Scale

1 Mild
2 Moderate
3 Severe
4 Very Severe
5 Worst Possible

Mark the area where the pain occurs with the number which corresponds to the intensity of the pain.

### In general, today I felt:

☐ Good
☐ Fair
☐ Poor

# Today's Conditions and Symptoms

Check the areas which apply and explain your conditions
& symptoms in the space provided. See the *Symptoms
Glossary* to help you describe your conditions.

☐ *Ears / Eyes / Nose*

_____

☐ *Mouth / Throat*

_____

☐ *Head / Neck / Back*

_____

☐ *Shoulders / Arms / Hands*

_____

☐ *Chest / Heart*

_____

☐ *Respiratory System*

_____

☐ *Digestive System*

_____

☐ *Hips / Legs / Feet*

_____

☐ *Male / Female Organs*

_____

☐ *Skin*

_____

☐ *Mood*

_____

☐ *Other*

_____

## Comments

_____
_____
_____

MemoryMinder©

# Today's Diet

In columns A&B, list the nutritional
facts you wish to monitor (i.e. fat,
calories, sodium, sugar, protein, etc.)

☐ **Breakfast**    A    B

Breakfast Totals

☐ **Lunch**

Lunch Totals

☐ **Dinner**

Dinner Totals

☐ **Snacks**

Snack Totals

GRAND TOTALS FOR TODAY:

A _____    B _____

_____  _____
Date                 Day

| | AM | PM |
|---|---|---|
| Weight | | |
| Temperature | | |
| Blood Pressure | | |
| Sugar Level | | |
| Hours slept last night | Number of hours: | Sound ☐ Restless ☐ |
| Naps taken today | How many? | Total hours: |

## *Today's Weather*

☐ Hot    ☐ Sunny    ☐ Damp
☐ Warm   ☐ Cloudy   ☐ Rainy
☐ Cool   ☐ Overcast ☐ Snowy
☐ Cold   ☐ Foggy    ☐ Windy

## *Drugs / Medications*

| Qty | | Description | Strength |
|---|---|---|---|
| AM | PM | | |
| | | | |
| | | | |
| | | | |
| | | | |
| | | | |
| | | | |

## *Vitamins / Herbs*

| Qty | | Description | Strengt |
|---|---|---|---|
| AM | PM | | |
| | | | |
| | | | |
| | | | |
| | | | |
| | | | |
| | | | |

MemoryMinder©

## *Physical Activity*

| Activity | Hours | Mins |
|---|---|---|
| | | |
| | | |
| | | |

## *Pain / Discomfort / Skin Changes*

### Scale

1 Mild
2 Moderate
3 Severe
4 Very Severe
5 Worst Possible

Mark the area where the pain occurs with the number which corresponds to the intensity of the pain.

## *In general, today I felt:*

☐ Good
☐ Fair
☐ Poor

## Today's Conditions and Symptoms

Check the areas which apply and explain your conditions or symptoms in the space provided. See the *Symptoms Glossary* to help you describe your conditions.

- [ ] *Ears / Eyes / Nose*
  _____
  _____

- [ ] *Mouth / Throat*
  _____
  _____

- [ ] *Head / Neck / Back*
  _____
  _____

- [ ] *Shoulders / Arms / Hands*
  _____
  _____

- [ ] *Chest / Heart*
  _____
  _____

- [ ] *Respiratory System*
  _____
  _____

- [ ] *Digestive System*
  _____
  _____

- [ ] *Hips / Legs / Feet*
  _____
  _____

- [ ] *Male / Female Organs*
  _____
  _____

- [ ] *Skin*
  _____
  _____

- [ ] *Mood*
  _____
  _____

- [ ] *Other*
  _____
  _____
  _____

## Comments

_____
_____
_____
_____

## Today's Diet

In columns A&B, list the nutritional facts you wish to monitor (i.e. fat, calories, sodium, sugar, protein, etc.)

| [ ] **Breakfast** | A | B |
|---|---|---|
| | | |
| | | |
| | | |
| | | |
| | | |
| Breakfast Totals | | |

| [ ] **Lunch** | | |
|---|---|---|
| | | |
| | | |
| | | |
| | | |
| | | |
| Lunch Totals | | |

| [ ] **Dinner** | | |
|---|---|---|
| | | |
| | | |
| | | |
| | | |
| | | |
| Dinner Totals | | |

| [ ] **Snacks** | | |
|---|---|---|
| | | |
| | | |
| | | |
| Snack Totals | | |

GRAND TOTALS FOR TODAY:

| A | B |
|---|---|
| | |

MemoryMinder©

_____  _____
Date                     Day

| | AM | PM |
|---|---|---|
| Weight | | |
| Temperature | | |
| Blood Pressure | / | / |
| Sugar Level | | |
| Hours slept last night | Number of hours: | Sound ☐ Restless ☐ |
| Naps taken today | How many? | Total hours: |

## Today's Weather

☐ Hot      ☐ Sunny      ☐ Damp
☐ Warm     ☐ Cloudy     ☐ Rainy
☐ Cool     ☐ Overcast   ☐ Snowy
☐ Cold     ☐ Foggy      ☐ Windy

## Drugs / Medications

| Qty | | Description | Strength |
|---|---|---|---|
| AM | PM | | |
| | | | |
| | | | |
| | | | |
| | | | |
| | | | |
| | | | |

## Vitamins / Herbs

| Qty | | Description | Strength |
|---|---|---|---|
| AM | PM | | |
| | | | |
| | | | |
| | | | |
| | | | |
| | | | |
| | | | |

MemoryMinder©

## Physical Activity

| Activity | Hours | Mins. |
|---|---|---|
| | | |
| | | |
| | | |

## Pain / Discomfort / Skin Changes

### Scale
1 Mild
2 Moderate
3 Severe
4 Very Severe
5 Worst Possible

Mark the area where the pain occurs with the number which corresponds to the intensity of the pain.

### In general, today I felt:

☐ Good
☐ Fair
☐ Poor

## Today's Conditions and Symptoms

Check the areas which apply and explain your conditions or symptoms in the space provided. See the *Symptoms Glossary* to help you describe your conditions.

☐ *Ears / Eyes / Nose*
_____
_____

☐ *Mouth / Throat*
_____
_____

☐ *Head / Neck / Back*
_____
_____

☐ *Shoulders / Arms / Hands*
_____
_____

☐ *Chest / Heart*
_____
_____

☐ *Respiratory System*
_____
_____

☐ *Digestive System*
_____
_____

☐ *Hips / Legs / Feet*
_____
_____

☐ *Male / Female Organs*
_____
_____

☐ *Skin*
_____
_____

☐ *Mood*
_____
_____

☐ *Other*
_____
_____
_____

## Comments
_____
_____
_____
_____

## Today's Diet

In columns A&B, list the nutritional facts you wish to monitor (i.e. fat, calories, sodium, sugar, protein, etc.)

| ☐ **Breakfast** | A | B |
|---|---|---|
|  |  |  |
|  |  |  |
|  |  |  |
|  |  |  |
|  |  |  |
| Breakfast Totals |  |  |

| ☐ **Lunch** |  |  |
|---|---|---|
|  |  |  |
|  |  |  |
|  |  |  |
|  |  |  |
|  |  |  |
| Lunch Totals |  |  |

| ☐ **Dinner** |  |  |
|---|---|---|
|  |  |  |
|  |  |  |
|  |  |  |
|  |  |  |
|  |  |  |
| Dinner Totals |  |  |

| ☐ **Snacks** |  |  |
|---|---|---|
|  |  |  |
|  |  |  |
|  |  |  |
| Snack Totals |  |  |

GRAND TOTALS FOR TODAY:

| A | B |
|---|---|
|  |  |

MemoryMinder©

_____  _____
Date              Day

| | AM | PM |
|---|---|---|
| Weight | | |
| Temperature | | |
| Blood Pressure | | |
| Sugar Level | | |
| Hours slept last night | Number of hours: | Sound ☐ Restless ☐ |
| Naps taken today | How many? | Total hours: |

## *Today's Weather*

☐ Hot     ☐ Sunny     ☐ Damp
☐ Warm    ☐ Cloudy    ☐ Rainy
☐ Cool    ☐ Overcast  ☐ Snowy
☐ Cold    ☐ Foggy     ☐ Windy

## *Drugs / Medications*

| Qty | | Description | Strength |
|---|---|---|---|
| AM | PM | | |
| | | | |
| | | | |
| | | | |
| | | | |
| | | | |
| | | | |

## *Vitamins / Herbs*

| Qty | | Description | Strength |
|---|---|---|---|
| AM | PM | | |
| | | | |
| | | | |
| | | | |
| | | | |
| | | | |
| | | | |

MemoryMinder©

## *Physical Activity*

| Activity | Hours | Mins. |
|---|---|---|
| | | |
| | | |
| | | |

## *Pain / Discomfort / Skin Changes*

### Scale

1 Mild
2 Moderate
3 Severe
4 Very Severe
5 Worst Possible

Mark the area where the pain occurs with the number which corresponds to the intensity of the pain.

### *In general, today I felt:*

☐ Good
☐ Fair
☐ Poor

# Today's Conditions and Symptoms

Check the areas which apply and explain your conditions symptoms in the space provided. See the *Symptoms Glossary* to help you describe your conditions.

☐ *Ears / Eyes / Nose*
_____

☐ *Mouth / Throat*
_____

☐ *Head / Neck / Back*
_____

☐ *Shoulders / Arms / Hands*
_____

☐ *Chest / Heart*
_____

☐ *Respiratory System*
_____

☐ *Digestive System*
_____

☐ *Hips / Legs / Feet*
_____

☐ *Male / Female Organs*
_____

☐ *Skin*
_____

☐ *Mood*
_____

☐ *Other*
_____
_____

## Comments
_____
_____
_____
_____

MemoryMinder©

## Today's Diet

In columns A&B, list the nutritional facts you wish to monitor (i.e. fat, calories, sodium, sugar, protein, etc.)

| ☐ **Breakfast** | A | B |
|---|---|---|
| | | |
| | | |
| | | |
| | | |
| | | |
| Breakfast Totals | | |

| ☐ **Lunch** | | |
|---|---|---|
| | | |
| | | |
| | | |
| | | |
| | | |
| Lunch Totals | | |

| ☐ **Dinner** | | |
|---|---|---|
| | | |
| | | |
| | | |
| | | |
| | | |
| Dinner Totals | | |

| ☐ **Snacks** | | |
|---|---|---|
| | | |
| | | |
| | | |
| Snack Totals | | |

GRAND TOTALS FOR TODAY:

| A | B |
|---|---|
| | |

|  | Date | Day |
|--|------|-----|

## Today's Weather

- [ ] Hot
- [ ] Warm
- [ ] Cool
- [ ] Cold
- [ ] Sunny
- [ ] Cloudy
- [ ] Overcast
- [ ] Foggy
- [ ] Damp
- [ ] Rainy
- [ ] Snowy
- [ ] Windy

|  | AM | PM |
|--|-----|-----|
| Weight | | |
| Temperature | | |
| Blood Pressure | | |
| Sugar Level | | |
| Hours slept last night | Number of hours: | Sound ☐ Restless ☐ |
| Naps taken today | How many? | Total hours: |

## Drugs / Medications

| Qty | | Description | Strength |
|-----|-----|-------------|----------|
| AM | PM | | |
| | | | |
| | | | |
| | | | |
| | | | |
| | | | |
| | | | |
| | | | |

MemoryMinder©

## Vitamins / Herbs

| Qty | | Description | Strengt |
|-----|-----|-------------|----------|
| AM | PM | | |
| | | | |
| | | | |
| | | | |
| | | | |
| | | | |
| | | | |
| | | | |

## Physical Activity

| Activity | Hours | Mins. |
|----------|-------|-------|
| | | |
| | | |
| | | |

## Pain / Discomfort / Skin Changes

### Scale

1 Mild
2 Moderate
3 Severe
4 Very Severe
5 Worst Possible

Mark the area where the pain occurs with the number which corresponds to the intensity of the pain.

### In general, today I felt:

- [ ] Good
- [ ] Fair
- [ ] Poor

# Today's Conditions and Symptoms

Check the areas which apply and explain your conditions
symptoms in the space provided. See the *Symptoms
Glossary* to help you describe your conditions.

☐ *Ears / Eyes / Nose*

_____

☐ *Mouth / Throat*

_____

☐ *Head / Neck / Back*

_____

☐ *Shoulders / Arms / Hands*

_____

☐ *Chest / Heart*

_____

☐ *Respiratory System*

_____

☐ *Digestive System*

_____

☐ *Hips / Legs / Feet*

_____

☐ *Male / Female Organs*

_____

☐ *Skin*

_____

☐ *Mood*

_____

☐ *Other*

_____

## Comments

_____
_____
_____
_____

# Today's Diet

In columns A&B, list the nutritional
facts you wish to monitor (i.e. fat,
calories, sodium, sugar, protein, etc.)

☐ *Breakfast*            A      B

Breakfast Totals

☐ *Lunch*

Lunch Totals

☐ *Dinner*

Dinner Totals

☐ *Snacks*

Snack Totals

GRAND TOTALS FOR TODAY:

| A | B |
|---|---|
|   |   |

MemoryMinder©

_____ _____
Date             Day

| | AM | PM |
|---|---|---|
| Weight | | |
| Temperature | | |
| Blood Pressure | | |
| Sugar Level | | |
| Hours slept last night | Number of hours: | Sound ☐ Restless ☐ |
| Naps taken today | How many? | Total hours: |

## Today's Weather

☐ Hot       ☐ Sunny       ☐ Damp
☐ Warm      ☐ Cloudy      ☐ Rainy
☐ Cool      ☐ Overcast    ☐ Snowy
☐ Cold      ☐ Foggy       ☐ Windy

## Drugs / Medications

| Qty | | Description | Strength |
|---|---|---|---|
| AM | PM | | |
| | | | |
| | | | |
| | | | |
| | | | |
| | | | |
| | | | |

## Vitamins / Herbs

| Qty | | Description | Strengt |
|---|---|---|---|
| AM | PM | | |
| | | | |
| | | | |
| | | | |
| | | | |
| | | | |
| | | | |

MemoryMinder©

## Physical Activity

| Activity | Hours | Mins |
|---|---|---|
| | | |
| | | |
| | | |

## Pain / Discomfort / Skin Changes

### Scale

1 Mild
2 Moderate
3 Severe
4 Very Severe
5 Worst Possible

Mark the area where the pain occurs with the number which corresponds to the intensity of the pain.

### In general, today I felt:

☐ Good
☐ Fair
☐ Poor

## Today's Conditions and Symptoms

Check the areas which apply and explain your conditions or symptoms in the space provided. See the *Symptoms Glossary* to help you describe your conditions.

☐ *Ears / Eyes / Nose*
_____

☐ *Mouth / Throat*
_____

☐ *Head / Neck / Back*
_____

☐ *Shoulders / Arms / Hands*
_____

☐ *Chest / Heart*
_____

☐ *Respiratory System*
_____

☐ *Digestive System*
_____

☐ *Hips / Legs / Feet*
_____

☐ *Male / Female Organs*
_____

☐ *Skin*
_____

☐ *Mood*
_____

☐ *Other*
_____
_____

### Comments
_____
_____
_____
_____

---

## Today's Diet

In columns A&B, list the nutritional facts you wish to monitor (i.e. fat, calories, sodium, sugar, protein, etc.)

| ☐ **Breakfast** | A | B |
|---|---|---|
| | | |
| | | |
| | | |
| | | |
| | | |
| | | |
| Breakfast Totals | | |

| ☐ **Lunch** | | |
|---|---|---|
| | | |
| | | |
| | | |
| | | |
| | | |
| | | |
| Lunch Totals | | |

| ☐ **Dinner** | | |
|---|---|---|
| | | |
| | | |
| | | |
| | | |
| | | |
| | | |
| Dinner Totals | | |

| ☐ **Snacks** | | |
|---|---|---|
| | | |
| | | |
| | | |
| Snack Totals | | |

| GRAND TOTALS FOR TODAY: | |
|---|---|
| A | B |

MemoryMinder©

| | | AM | PM |
|---|---|---|---|
| _____ _____ | Weight | | |
| Date          Day | Temperature | | |
| | Blood Pressure | | |
| | Sugar Level | | |

## Today's Weather

- [ ] Hot
- [ ] Warm
- [ ] Cool
- [ ] Cold
- [ ] Sunny
- [ ] Cloudy
- [ ] Overcast
- [ ] Foggy
- [ ] Damp
- [ ] Rainy
- [ ] Snowy
- [ ] Windy

| | AM | PM |
|---|---|---|
| Weight | | |
| Temperature | | |
| Blood Pressure | | |
| Sugar Level | | |
| Hours slept last night | Number of hours: | Sound ☐ Restless ☐ |
| Naps taken today | How many? | Total hours: |

## Drugs / Medications

| Qty | | Description | Strength |
|---|---|---|---|
| AM | PM | | |
| | | | |
| | | | |
| | | | |
| | | | |
| | | | |
| | | | |

## Vitamins / Herbs

| Qty | | Description | Strengt |
|---|---|---|---|
| AM | PM | | |
| | | | |
| | | | |
| | | | |
| | | | |
| | | | |
| | | | |

MemoryMinder©

## Physical Activity

| Activity | Hours | Mins |
|---|---|---|
| | | |
| | | |
| | | |

## Pain / Discomfort / Skin Changes

### Scale

1 Mild
2 Moderate
3 Severe
4 Very Severe
5 Worst Possible

Mark the area where the pain occurs with the number which corresponds to the intensity of the pain.

### In general, today I felt:

- [ ] Good
- [ ] Fair
- [ ] Poor

## Today's Conditions and Symptoms

Check the areas which apply and explain your conditions or symptoms in the space provided. See the *Symptoms Glossary* to help you describe your conditions.

☐ *Ears / Eyes / Nose*
_____
_____

☐ *Mouth / Throat*
_____
_____

☐ *Head / Neck / Back*
_____
_____

☐ *Shoulders / Arms / Hands*
_____
_____

☐ *Chest / Heart*
_____
_____

☐ *Respiratory System*
_____
_____

☐ *Digestive System*
_____
_____

☐ *Hips / Legs / Feet*
_____
_____

☐ *Male / Female Organs*
_____
_____

☐ *Skin*
_____
_____

☐ *Mood*
_____
_____

☐ *Other*
_____
_____
_____

## Comments
_____
_____
_____
_____

## Today's Diet

In columns A&B, list the nutritional facts you wish to monitor (i.e. fat, calories, sodium, sugar, protein, etc.)

| ☐ **Breakfast** | A | B |
| --- | --- | --- |
| | | |
| | | |
| | | |
| | | |
| | | |
| Breakfast Totals | | |

| ☐ **Lunch** | | |
| --- | --- | --- |
| | | |
| | | |
| | | |
| | | |
| | | |
| Lunch Totals | | |

| ☐ **Dinner** | | |
| --- | --- | --- |
| | | |
| | | |
| | | |
| | | |
| | | |
| Dinner Totals | | |

| ☐ **Snacks** | | |
| --- | --- | --- |
| | | |
| | | |
| | | |
| Snack Totals | | |

GRAND TOTALS FOR TODAY:

| A | B |
| --- | --- |
| | |

MemoryMinder©

|  | | AM | PM |
|---|---|---|---|
| **Date** _____ **Day** _____ | | | |
| Weight | | | |
| Temperature | | | |
| Blood Pressure | | | |
| Sugar Level | | | |
| Hours slept last night | | Number of hours: | Sound ☐ Restless ☐ |
| Naps taken today | | How many? | Total hours: |

## Today's Weather

☐ Hot    ☐ Sunny    ☐ Damp
☐ Warm    ☐ Cloudy    ☐ Rainy
☐ Cool    ☐ Overcast    ☐ Snowy
☐ Cold    ☐ Foggy    ☐ Windy

## Drugs / Medications

| Qty AM | PM | Description | Strength |
|---|---|---|---|
|  |  |  |  |
|  |  |  |  |
|  |  |  |  |
|  |  |  |  |
|  |  |  |  |
|  |  |  |  |
|  |  |  |  |

## Vitamins / Herbs

| Qty AM | PM | Description | Strength |
|---|---|---|---|
|  |  |  |  |
|  |  |  |  |
|  |  |  |  |
|  |  |  |  |
|  |  |  |  |
|  |  |  |  |
|  |  |  |  |

MemoryMinder©

## Physical Activity

| Activity | Hours | Mins |
|---|---|---|
|  |  |  |
|  |  |  |
|  |  |  |
|  |  |  |

## Pain / Discomfort / Skin Changes

### Scale

1 Mild
2 Moderate
3 Severe
4 Very Severe
5 Worst Possible

Mark the area where the pain occurs with the number which corresponds to the intensity of the pain.

### In general, today I felt:

☐ Good
☐ Fair
☐ Poor

## Today's Conditions and Symptoms

Check the areas which apply and explain your conditions or symptoms in the space provided. See the *Symptoms Glossary* to help you describe your conditions.

☐ *Ears / Eyes / Nose*

_____

☐ *Mouth / Throat*

_____

☐ *Head / Neck / Back*

_____

☐ *Shoulders / Arms / Hands*

_____

☐ *Chest / Heart*

_____

☐ *Respiratory System*

_____

☐ *Digestive System*

_____

☐ *Hips / Legs / Feet*

_____

☐ *Male / Female Organs*

_____

☐ *Skin*

_____

☐ *Mood*

_____

☐ *Other*

_____
_____

## Comments

_____
_____
_____
_____

## Today's Diet

In columns A&B, list the nutritional facts you wish to monitor (i.e. fat, calories, sodium, sugar, protein, etc.)

| ☐ **Breakfast** | A | B |
|---|---|---|
| | | |
| | | |
| | | |
| | | |
| Breakfast Totals | | |

| ☐ **Lunch** | | |
|---|---|---|
| | | |
| | | |
| | | |
| | | |
| | | |
| Lunch Totals | | |

| ☐ **Dinner** | | |
|---|---|---|
| | | |
| | | |
| | | |
| | | |
| | | |
| Dinner Totals | | |

| ☐ **Snacks** | | |
|---|---|---|
| | | |
| | | |
| | | |
| Snack Totals | | |

GRAND TOTALS FOR TODAY:

| A | B |
|---|---|
| | |

MemoryMinder©

_____ _____
Date                Day

| | | AM | PM |
|---|---|---|---|
| Weight | | | |
| Temperature | | | |
| Blood Pressure | | | |
| Sugar Level | | | |
| Hours slept last night | | Number of hours: | Sound ☐ Restless |
| Naps taken today | | How many? | Total hours: |

## Today's Weather

☐ Hot     ☐ Sunny      ☐ Damp
☐ Warm    ☐ Cloudy     ☐ Rainy
☐ Cool    ☐ Overcast   ☐ Snowy
☐ Cold    ☐ Foggy      ☐ Windy

## Drugs / Medications

| Qty | | Description | Strength |
|---|---|---|---|
| AM | PM | | |
| | | | |
| | | | |
| | | | |
| | | | |
| | | | |
| | | | |

## Vitamins / Herbs

| Qty | | Description | Strength |
|---|---|---|---|
| AM | PM | | |
| | | | |
| | | | |
| | | | |
| | | | |
| | | | |

MemoryMinder©

## Physical Activity

| Activity | Hours | Mins. |
|---|---|---|
| | | |
| | | |
| | | |

## Pain / Discomfort / Skin Changes

### Scale

1 Mild
2 Moderate
3 Severe
4 Very Severe
5 Worst Possible

Mark the area where the pain occurs with the number which corresponds to the intensity of the pain.

### In general, today I felt:

☐ Good
☐ Fair
☐ Poor

## Today's Conditions and Symptoms

Check the areas which apply and explain your conditions or symptoms in the space provided. See the *Symptoms Glossary* to help you describe your conditions.

☐ *Ears / Eyes / Nose*

_____

☐ *Mouth / Throat*

_____

☐ *Head / Neck / Back*

_____

☐ *Shoulders / Arms / Hands*

_____

☐ *Chest / Heart*

_____

☐ *Respiratory System*

_____

☐ *Digestive System*

_____

☐ *Hips / Legs / Feet*

_____

☐ *Male / Female Organs*

_____

☐ *Skin*

_____

☐ *Mood*

_____

☐ *Other*

_____
_____

## Comments

_____
_____
_____
_____

MemoryMinder©

## Today's Diet

In columns A&B, list the nutritional facts you wish to monitor (i.e. fat, calories, sodium, sugar, protein, etc.)

☐ *Breakfast*

| | A | B |
|---|---|---|
| | | |
| | | |
| | | |
| | | |
| | | |
| Breakfast Totals | | |

☐ *Lunch*

| | A | B |
|---|---|---|
| | | |
| | | |
| | | |
| | | |
| | | |
| Lunch Totals | | |

☐ *Dinner*

| | A | B |
|---|---|---|
| | | |
| | | |
| | | |
| | | |
| | | |
| Dinner Totals | | |

☐ *Snacks*

| | A | B |
|---|---|---|
| | | |
| | | |
| | | |
| Snack Totals | | |

GRAND TOTALS FOR TODAY:

| A | B |
|---|---|
| | |

| | | AM | PM |
|---|---|---|---|
| Weight | | | |
| Temperature | | | |
| Blood Pressure | | | |
| Sugar Level | | | |
| Hours slept last night | | Number of hours: | Sound ☐ Restless ☐ |
| Naps taken today | | How many? | Total hours: |

_____  _____
Date                        Day

## Today's Weather

☐ Hot      ☐ Sunny      ☐ Damp
☐ Warm    ☐ Cloudy     ☐ Rainy
☐ Cool     ☐ Overcast   ☐ Snowy
☐ Cold     ☐ Foggy      ☐ Windy

## Drugs / Medications

| Qty | | Description | Strength |
|---|---|---|---|
| AM | PM | | |
| | | | |
| | | | |
| | | | |
| | | | |
| | | | |
| | | | |
| | | | |

## Vitamins / Herbs

| Qty | | Description | Strength |
|---|---|---|---|
| AM | PM | | |
| | | | |
| | | | |
| | | | |
| | | | |
| | | | |
| | | | |
| | | | |

MemoryMinder©

## Physical Activity

| Activity | Hours | Mins. |
|---|---|---|
| | | |
| | | |
| | | |
| | | |

## Pain / Discomfort / Skin Changes

### Scale

1 Mild
2 Moderate
3 Severe
4 Very Severe
5 Worst Possible

Mark the area where the pain occurs with the number which corresponds to the intensity of the pain.

### In general, today I felt:

☐ Good
☐ Fair
☐ Poor

# Today's Conditions and Symptoms

Check the areas which apply and explain your conditions
or symptoms in the space provided. See the *Symptoms
Glossary* to help you describe your conditions.

☐ **Ears / Eyes / Nose**
_____

☐ **Mouth / Throat**
_____

☐ **Head / Neck / Back**
_____

☐ **Shoulders / Arms / Hands**
_____

☐ **Chest / Heart**
_____

☐ **Respiratory System**
_____

☐ **Digestive System**
_____

☐ **Hips / Legs / Feet**
_____

☐ **Male / Female Organs**
_____

☐ **Skin**
_____

☐ **Mood**
_____

☐ **Other**
_____
_____

## Comments
_____
_____
_____

MemoryMinder©

# Today's Diet

In columns A&B, list the nutritional
facts you wish to monitor (i.e. fat,
calories, sodium, sugar, protein, etc.)

☐ **Breakfast**    A    B

Breakfast Totals

☐ **Lunch**

Lunch Totals

☐ **Dinner**

Dinner Totals

☐ **Snacks**

Snack Totals

GRAND TOTALS FOR TODAY:

A _____    B _____

_____  _____
Date              Day

|  | AM | PM |
|---|---|---|
| Weight | | |
| Temperature | | |
| Blood Pressure | | |
| Sugar Level | | |
| Hours slept last night | Number of hours: | Sound ☐ Restless ☐ |
| Naps taken today | How many? | Total hours: |

## Today's Weather

☐ Hot        ☐ Sunny       ☐ Damp
☐ Warm     ☐ Cloudy     ☐ Rainy
☐ Cool       ☐ Overcast  ☐ Snowy
☐ Cold       ☐ Foggy      ☐ Windy

## Drugs / Medications

| Qty | | Description | Strength |
|---|---|---|---|
| AM | PM | | |
| | | | |
| | | | |
| | | | |
| | | | |
| | | | |
| | | | |

## Vitamins / Herbs

| Qty | | Description | Strength |
|---|---|---|---|
| AM | PM | | |
| | | | |
| | | | |
| | | | |
| | | | |
| | | | |
| | | | |

MemoryMinder©

## Physical Activity

| Activity | Hours | Mins. |
|---|---|---|
| | | |
| | | |
| | | |

## Pain / Discomfort / Skin Changes

### Scale

1 Mild
2 Moderate
3 Severe
4 Very Severe
5 Worst Possible

Mark the area where the pain occurs with the number which corresponds to the intensity of the pain.

## In general, today I felt:

☐ Good
☐ Fair
☐ Poor

## Today's Conditions and Symptoms

Check the areas which apply and explain your conditions or symptoms in the space provided. See the *Symptoms Glossary* to help you describe your conditions.

☐ *Ears / Eyes / Nose*

_____

☐ *Mouth / Throat*

_____

☐ *Head / Neck / Back*

_____

☐ *Shoulders / Arms / Hands*

_____

☐ *Chest / Heart*

_____

☐ *Respiratory System*

_____

☐ *Digestive System*

_____

☐ *Hips / Legs / Feet*

_____

☐ *Male / Female Organs*

_____

☐ *Skin*

_____

☐ *Mood*

_____

☐ *Other*

_____

## Comments

_____
_____
_____
_____

## Today's Diet

In columns A&B, list the nutritional facts you wish to monitor (i.e. fat, calories, sodium, sugar, protein, etc.)

☐ **Breakfast**

| | A | B |
|---|---|---|
| | | |
| | | |
| | | |
| | | |
| | | |
| Breakfast Totals | | |

☐ **Lunch**

| | A | B |
|---|---|---|
| | | |
| | | |
| | | |
| | | |
| | | |
| Lunch Totals | | |

☐ **Dinner**

| | A | B |
|---|---|---|
| | | |
| | | |
| | | |
| | | |
| | | |
| Dinner Totals | | |

☐ **Snacks**

| | A | B |
|---|---|---|
| | | |
| | | |
| | | |
| Snack Totals | | |

GRAND TOTALS FOR TODAY:

| A | B |
|---|---|
| | |

MemoryMinder©

| | | AM | PM |
|---|---|---|---|
| Weight | | | |
| Temperature | | | |
| Blood Pressure | | | |
| Sugar Level | | | |
| Hours slept last night | Number of hours: | | Sound ☐ Restless ☐ |
| Naps taken today | How many? | | Total hours: |

_____ _____
Date            Day

## Today's Weather

☐ Hot          ☐ Sunny          ☐ Damp
☐ Warm        ☐ Cloudy         ☐ Rainy
☐ Cool         ☐ Overcast       ☐ Snowy
☐ Cold         ☐ Foggy          ☐ Windy

## Drugs / Medications

| Qty AM | Qty PM | Description | Strength |
|---|---|---|---|
| | | | |
| | | | |
| | | | |
| | | | |
| | | | |
| | | | |
| | | | |

## Vitamins / Herbs

| Qty AM | Qty PM | Description | Strength |
|---|---|---|---|
| | | | |
| | | | |
| | | | |
| | | | |
| | | | |
| | | | |
| | | | |

MemoryMinder©

## Physical Activity

| Activity | Hours | Mins. |
|---|---|---|
| | | |
| | | |
| | | |

## Pain / Discomfort / Skin Changes

### Scale

1 Mild
2 Moderate
3 Severe
4 Very Severe
5 Worst Possible

Mark the area where the pain occurs with the number which corresponds to the intensity of the pain.

### In general, today I felt:

☐ Good
☐ Fair
☐ Poor

## Today's Conditions and Symptoms

Check the areas which apply and explain your conditions or symptoms in the space provided. See the *Symptoms Glossary* to help you describe your conditions.

☐ *Ears / Eyes / Nose*
_____
_____

☐ *Mouth / Throat*
_____
_____

☐ *Head / Neck / Back*
_____
_____

☐ *Shoulders / Arms / Hands*
_____
_____

☐ *Chest / Heart*
_____
_____

☐ *Respiratory System*
_____
_____

☐ *Digestive System*
_____
_____

☐ *Hips / Legs / Feet*
_____
_____

☐ *Male / Female Organs*
_____
_____

☐ *Skin*
_____
_____

☐ *Mood*
_____
_____

☐ *Other*
_____
_____

## Comments
_____
_____
_____
_____
_____

## Today's Diet

In columns A&B, list the nutritional facts you wish to monitor (i.e. fat, calories, sodium, sugar, protein, etc.)

| ☐ **Breakfast** | A | B |
| --- | --- | --- |
| | | |
| | | |
| | | |
| | | |
| | | |
| Breakfast Totals | | |

| ☐ **Lunch** | | |
| --- | --- | --- |
| | | |
| | | |
| | | |
| | | |
| | | |
| Lunch Totals | | |

| ☐ **Dinner** | | |
| --- | --- | --- |
| | | |
| | | |
| | | |
| | | |
| | | |
| Dinner Totals | | |

| ☐ **Snacks** | | |
| --- | --- | --- |
| | | |
| | | |
| | | |
| Snack Totals | | |

GRAND TOTALS FOR TODAY:

| A | B |
| --- | --- |
| | |

MemoryMinder©

| | Date | Day |
|---|---|---|

| | AM | PM |
|---|---|---|
| Weight | | |
| Temperature | | |
| Blood Pressure | | |
| Sugar Level | | |
| Hours slept last night | Number of hours: | Sound ☐ Restless ☐ |
| Naps taken today | How many? | Total hours: |

## Today's Weather

☐ Hot    ☐ Sunny    ☐ Damp
☐ Warm    ☐ Cloudy    ☐ Rainy
☐ Cool    ☐ Overcast    ☐ Snowy
☐ Cold    ☐ Foggy    ☐ Windy

## Drugs / Medications

| Qty | | Description | Strength |
|---|---|---|---|
| AM | PM | | |
| | | | |
| | | | |
| | | | |
| | | | |
| | | | |
| | | | |

## Vitamins / Herbs

| Qty | | Description | Strength |
|---|---|---|---|
| AM | PM | | |
| | | | |
| | | | |
| | | | |
| | | | |
| | | | |
| | | | |

MemoryMinder©

## Physical Activity

| Activity | Hours | Mins. |
|---|---|---|
| | | |
| | | |
| | | |
| | | |

## Pain / Discomfort / Skin Changes

### Scale

1 Mild
2 Moderate
3 Severe
4 Very Severe
5 Worst Possible

Mark the area where the pain occurs with the number which corresponds to the intensity of the pain.

### In general, today I felt:

☐ Good
☐ Fair
☐ Poor

## Today's Conditions and Symptoms

Check the areas which apply and explain your conditions or symptoms in the space provided. See the *Symptoms Glossary* to help you describe your conditions.

☐ *Ears / Eyes / Nose*

_____

☐ *Mouth / Throat*

_____

☐ *Head / Neck / Back*

_____

☐ *Shoulders / Arms / Hands*

_____

☐ *Chest / Heart*

_____

☐ *Respiratory System*

_____

☐ *Digestive System*

_____

☐ *Hips / Legs / Feet*

_____

☐ *Male / Female Organs*

_____

☐ *Skin*

_____

☐ *Mood*

_____

☐ *Other*

_____

_____

## Comments

_____
_____
_____
_____
_____

## Today's Diet

In columns A&B, list the nutritional facts you wish to monitor (i.e. fat, calories, sodium, sugar, protein, etc.)

☐ **Breakfast**

| | A | B |
|---|---|---|
| | | |
| | | |
| | | |
| | | |
| | | |
| Breakfast Totals | | |

☐ **Lunch**

| | | |
|---|---|---|
| | | |
| | | |
| | | |
| | | |
| | | |
| Lunch Totals | | |

☐ **Dinner**

| | | |
|---|---|---|
| | | |
| | | |
| | | |
| | | |
| | | |
| Dinner Totals | | |

☐ **Snacks**

| | | |
|---|---|---|
| | | |
| | | |
| | | |
| Snack Totals | | |

GRAND TOTALS FOR TODAY:

| A | B |
|---|---|
| | |

MemoryMinder©

| | Date | | Day |
| --- | --- | --- | --- |

| | AM | PM |
| --- | --- | --- |
| Weight | | |
| Temperature | | |
| Blood Pressure | | |
| Sugar Level | | |
| Hours slept last night | Number of hours: | Sound ☐ Restless ☐ |
| Naps taken today | How many? | Total hours: |

## Today's Weather

☐ Hot    ☐ Sunny    ☐ Damp
☐ Warm   ☐ Cloudy   ☐ Rainy
☐ Cool   ☐ Overcast ☐ Snowy
☐ Cold   ☐ Foggy    ☐ Windy

## Drugs / Medications

| Qty | | Description | Strength |
| --- | --- | --- | --- |
| AM | PM | | |
| | | | |
| | | | |
| | | | |
| | | | |
| | | | |
| | | | |
| | | | |

## Vitamins / Herbs

| Qty | | Description | Strength |
| --- | --- | --- | --- |
| AM | PM | | |
| | | | |
| | | | |
| | | | |
| | | | |
| | | | |
| | | | |

MemoryMinder©

## Physical Activity

| Activity | Hours | Mins |
| --- | --- | --- |
| | | |
| | | |
| | | |

## Pain / Discomfort / Skin Changes

### Scale

1 Mild
2 Moderate
3 Severe
4 Very Severe
5 Worst Possible

Mark the area where the pain occurs with the number which corresponds to the intensity of the pain.

### In general, today I felt:

☐ Good
☐ Fair
☐ Poor

# Today's Conditions and Symptoms

Check the areas which apply and explain your conditions symptoms in the space provided. See the *Symptoms Glossary* to help you describe your conditions.

☐ *Ears / Eyes / Nose*

_____

☐ *Mouth / Throat*

_____

☐ *Head / Neck / Back*

_____

☐ *Shoulders / Arms / Hands*

_____

☐ *Chest / Heart*

_____

☐ *Respiratory System*

_____

☐ *Digestive System*

_____

☐ *Hips / Legs / Feet*

_____

☐ *Male / Female Organs*

_____

☐ *Skin*

_____

☐ *Mood*

_____

☐ *Other*

_____

## Comments

_____
_____
_____
_____

MemoryMinder©

# Today's Diet

In columns A&B, list the nutritional facts you wish to monitor (i.e. fat, calories, sodium, sugar, protein, etc.)

☐ **Breakfast**

| | A | B |
|---|---|---|
| | | |
| | | |
| | | |
| | | |
| Breakfast Totals | | |

☐ **Lunch**

| | A | B |
|---|---|---|
| | | |
| | | |
| | | |
| | | |
| Lunch Totals | | |

☐ **Dinner**

| | A | B |
|---|---|---|
| | | |
| | | |
| | | |
| | | |
| Dinner Totals | | |

☐ **Snacks**

| | A | B |
|---|---|---|
| | | |
| | | |
| Snack Totals | | |

GRAND TOTALS FOR TODAY:

| A | B |
|---|---|
| | |

_____  _____
Date           Day

| | AM | PM |
|---|---|---|
| Weight | | |
| Temperature | | |
| Blood Pressure | | |
| Sugar Level | | |
| Hours slept last night | Number of hours: | Sound ☐ Restless ☐ |
| Naps taken today | How many? | Total hours: |

## *Today's Weather*

☐ Hot      ☐ Sunny      ☐ Damp
☐ Warm     ☐ Cloudy     ☐ Rainy
☐ Cool     ☐ Overcast   ☐ Snowy
☐ Cold     ☐ Foggy      ☐ Windy

## *Drugs / Medications*

| Qty | | Description | Strength |
|---|---|---|---|
| AM | PM | | |
| | | | |
| | | | |
| | | | |
| | | | |
| | | | |
| | | | |

## *Vitamins / Herbs*

| Qty | | Description | Strengt |
|---|---|---|---|
| AM | PM | | |
| | | | |
| | | | |
| | | | |
| | | | |
| | | | |
| | | | |

MemoryMinder©

## *Physical Activity*

| Activity | Hours | Mins |
|---|---|---|
| | | |
| | | |
| | | |

## *Pain / Discomfort / Skin Changes*

### Scale

1 Mild
2 Moderate
3 Severe
4 Very Severe
5 Worst Possible

Mark the area where the pain occurs with the number which corresponds to the intensity of the pain.

### *In general, today I felt:*

☐ Good
☐ Fair
☐ Poor

# Today's Conditions and Symptoms

Check the areas which apply and explain your conditions / symptoms in the space provided. See the *Symptoms Glossary* to help you describe your conditions.

☐ *Ears / Eyes / Nose*
_____
_____

☐ *Mouth / Throat*
_____
_____

☐ *Head / Neck / Back*
_____
_____

☐ *Shoulders / Arms / Hands*
_____
_____

☐ *Chest / Heart*
_____
_____

☐ *Respiratory System*
_____
_____

☐ *Digestive System*
_____
_____

☐ *Hips / Legs / Feet*
_____
_____

☐ *Male / Female Organs*
_____
_____

☐ *Skin*
_____
_____

☐ *Mood*
_____
_____

☐ *Other*
_____
_____
_____

## Comments
_____
_____
_____
_____

## Today's Diet

In columns A&B, list the nutritional facts you wish to monitor (i.e. fat, calories, sodium, sugar, protein, etc.)

☐ **Breakfast**  A  B

Breakfast Totals

☐ **Lunch**

Lunch Totals

☐ **Dinner**

Dinner Totals

☐ **Snacks**

Snack Totals

GRAND TOTALS FOR TODAY:

| A | B |
|---|---|
|   |   |

MemoryMinder©

|  | Date | | Day |
| --- | --- | --- | --- |

|  | AM | PM |
| --- | --- | --- |
| Weight | | |
| Temperature | | |
| Blood Pressure | | |
| Sugar Level | | |
| Hours slept last night | Number of hours: | Sound ☐ Restless ☐ |
| Naps taken today | How many? | Total hours: |

## Today's Weather

☐ Hot    ☐ Sunny    ☐ Damp
☐ Warm    ☐ Cloudy    ☐ Rainy
☐ Cool    ☐ Overcast    ☐ Snowy
☐ Cold    ☐ Foggy    ☐ Windy

## Drugs / Medications

| Qty | | Description | Strength |
| --- | --- | --- | --- |
| AM | PM | | |
| | | | |
| | | | |
| | | | |
| | | | |
| | | | |
| | | | |

## Vitamins / Herbs

| Qty | | Description | Strength |
| --- | --- | --- | --- |
| AM | PM | | |
| | | | |
| | | | |
| | | | |
| | | | |
| | | | |
| | | | |

MemoryMinder©

## Physical Activity

| Activity | Hours | Mins. |
| --- | --- | --- |
| | | |
| | | |
| | | |

## Pain / Discomfort / Skin Changes

### Scale

1 Mild
2 Moderate
3 Severe
4 Very Severe
5 Worst Possible

Mark the area where the pain occurs with the number which corresponds to the intensity of the pain.

### In general, today I felt:

☐ Good
☐ Fair
☐ Poor

## Today's Conditions and Symptoms

Check the areas which apply and explain your conditions or symptoms in the space provided. See the *Symptoms Glossary* to help you describe your conditions.

☐ *Ears / Eyes / Nose*

_____

☐ *Mouth / Throat*

_____

☐ *Head / Neck / Back*

_____

☐ *Shoulders / Arms / Hands*

_____

☐ *Chest / Heart*

_____

☐ *Respiratory System*

_____

☐ *Digestive System*

_____

☐ *Hips / Legs / Feet*

_____

☐ *Male / Female Organs*

_____

☐ *Skin*

_____

☐ *Mood*

_____

☐ *Other*

_____
_____

## Comments

_____
_____
_____
_____

MemoryMinder©

## Today's Diet

In columns A&B, list the nutritional facts you wish to monitor (i.e. fat, calories, sodium, sugar, protein, etc.)

| ☐ Breakfast | A | B |
|---|---|---|
| | | |
| | | |
| | | |
| | | |
| Breakfast Totals | | |

| ☐ Lunch | | |
|---|---|---|
| | | |
| | | |
| | | |
| | | |
| | | |
| Lunch Totals | | |

| ☐ Dinner | | |
|---|---|---|
| | | |
| | | |
| | | |
| | | |
| | | |
| Dinner Totals | | |

| ☐ Snacks | | |
|---|---|---|
| | | |
| | | |
| | | |
| Snack Totals | | |

GRAND TOTALS FOR TODAY:

| A | | B | |
|---|---|---|---|
| | | | |

| | AM | PM |
|---|---|---|
| Weight | | |
| Temperature | | |
| Blood Pressure | | |
| Sugar Level | | |
| Hours slept last night | Number of hours: | Sound ☐ Restless ☐ |
| Naps taken today | How many? | Total hours: |

_____  _____
Date               Day

## Today's Weather

☐ Hot      ☐ Sunny       ☐ Damp
☐ Warm     ☐ Cloudy      ☐ Rainy
☐ Cool     ☐ Overcast    ☐ Snowy
☐ Cold     ☐ Foggy       ☐ Windy

## Drugs / Medications

| Qty | | Description | Strength |
|---|---|---|---|
| AM | PM | | |
| | | | |
| | | | |
| | | | |
| | | | |
| | | | |
| | | | |
| | | | |

## Vitamins / Herbs

| Qty | | Description | Strengt |
|---|---|---|---|
| AM | PM | | |
| | | | |
| | | | |
| | | | |
| | | | |
| | | | |
| | | | |
| | | | |

MemoryMinder©

## Physical Activity

| Activity | Hours | Mins. |
|---|---|---|
| | | |
| | | |
| | | |

## Pain / Discomfort / Skin Changes

### Scale

1 Mild
2 Moderate
3 Severe
4 Very Severe
5 Worst Possible

Mark the area where the pain occurs with the number which corresponds to the intensity of the pain.

### In general, today I felt:

☐ Good
☐ Fair
☐ Poor

# Today's Conditions and Symptoms

Check the areas which apply and explain your conditions
symptoms in the space provided. See the *Symptoms
Glossary* to help you describe your conditions.

☐ *Ears / Eyes / Nose*
_____

☐ *Mouth / Throat*
_____

☐ *Head / Neck / Back*
_____

☐ *Shoulders / Arms / Hands*
_____

☐ *Chest / Heart*
_____

☐ *Respiratory System*
_____

☐ *Digestive System*
_____

☐ *Hips / Legs / Feet*
_____

☐ *Male / Female Organs*
_____

☐ *Skin*
_____

☐ *Mood*
_____

☐ *Other*
_____
_____

## Comments
_____
_____
_____
_____

# Today's Diet

In columns A&B, list the nutritional
facts you wish to monitor (i.e. fat,
calories, sodium, sugar, protein, etc.)

| ☐ **Breakfast** | A | B |
|---|---|---|
| | | |
| | | |
| | | |
| | | |
| | | |
| Breakfast Totals | | |

| ☐ **Lunch** | | |
|---|---|---|
| | | |
| | | |
| | | |
| | | |
| | | |
| Lunch Totals | | |

| ☐ **Dinner** | | |
|---|---|---|
| | | |
| | | |
| | | |
| | | |
| | | |
| Dinner Totals | | |

| ☐ **Snacks** | | |
|---|---|---|
| | | |
| | | |
| | | |
| Snack Totals | | |

GRAND TOTALS FOR TODAY:

| A | B |
|---|---|
| | |

| | Date | | Day |
| --- | --- | --- | --- |

| | AM | PM |
| --- | --- | --- |
| Weight | | |
| Temperature | | |
| Blood Pressure | | |
| Sugar Level | | |
| Hours slept last night | Number of hours: | Sound ☐ Restless ☐ |
| Naps taken today | How many? | Total hours: |

## Today's Weather

☐ Hot  ☐ Sunny  ☐ Damp
☐ Warm  ☐ Cloudy  ☐ Rainy
☐ Cool  ☐ Overcast  ☐ Snowy
☐ Cold  ☐ Foggy  ☐ Windy

## Drugs / Medications

| Qty | | Description | Strength |
| --- | --- | --- | --- |
| AM | PM | | |
| | | | |
| | | | |
| | | | |
| | | | |
| | | | |
| | | | |

## Vitamins / Herbs

| Qty | | Description | Strength |
| --- | --- | --- | --- |
| AM | PM | | |
| | | | |
| | | | |
| | | | |
| | | | |
| | | | |
| | | | |

MemoryMinder©

## Physical Activity

| Activity | Hours | Mins. |
| --- | --- | --- |
| | | |
| | | |
| | | |
| | | |

## Pain / Discomfort / Skin Changes

### Scale

1 Mild
2 Moderate
3 Severe
4 Very Severe
5 Worst Possible

Mark the area where the pain occurs with the number which corresponds to the intensity of the pain.

### In general, today I felt:

☐ Good
☐ Fair
☐ Poor

## Today's Conditions and Symptoms

Check the areas which apply and explain your conditions or symptoms in the space provided. See the *Symptoms Glossary* to help you describe your conditions.

☐ *Ears / Eyes / Nose*

_____

☐ *Mouth / Throat*

_____

☐ *Head / Neck / Back*

_____

☐ *Shoulders / Arms / Hands*

_____

☐ *Chest / Heart*

_____

☐ *Respiratory System*

_____

☐ *Digestive System*

_____

☐ *Hips / Legs / Feet*

_____

☐ *Male / Female Organs*

_____

☐ *Skin*

_____

☐ *Mood*

_____

☐ *Other*

_____
_____

## Comments

_____
_____
_____
_____

MemoryMinder©

## Today's Diet

In columns A&B, list the nutritional facts you wish to monitor (i.e. fat, calories, sodium, sugar, protein, etc.)

| ☐ **Breakfast** | A | B |
|---|---|---|
| | | |
| | | |
| | | |
| | | |
| | | |
| Breakfast Totals | | |

| ☐ **Lunch** | | |
|---|---|---|
| | | |
| | | |
| | | |
| | | |
| | | |
| Lunch Totals | | |

| ☐ **Dinner** | | |
|---|---|---|
| | | |
| | | |
| | | |
| | | |
| | | |
| Dinner Totals | | |

| ☐ **Snacks** | | |
|---|---|---|
| | | |
| | | |
| | | |
| Snack Totals | | |

GRAND TOTALS FOR TODAY:

| A | B |
|---|---|
| | |

_____  _____
Date             Day

|  | AM | PM |
|---|---|---|
| Weight | | |
| Temperature | | |
| Blood Pressure | | |
| Sugar Level | | |
| Hours slept last night | Number of hours: | Sound ☐ Restless ☐ |
| Naps taken today | How many? | Total hours: |

## Today's Weather

☐ Hot       ☐ Sunny      ☐ Damp
☐ Warm      ☐ Cloudy     ☐ Rainy
☐ Cool      ☐ Overcast   ☐ Snowy
☐ Cold      ☐ Foggy      ☐ Windy

## Drugs / Medications

| Qty | | Description | Strength |
|---|---|---|---|
| AM | PM | | |
| | | | |
| | | | |
| | | | |
| | | | |
| | | | |
| | | | |

## Vitamins / Herbs

| Qty | | Description | Strength |
|---|---|---|---|
| AM | PM | | |
| | | | |
| | | | |
| | | | |
| | | | |
| | | | |
| | | | |

MemoryMinder©

## Physical Activity

| Activity | Hours | Mins. |
|---|---|---|
| | | |
| | | |
| | | |

## Pain / Discomfort / Skin Changes

### Scale

1 Mild
2 Moderate
3 Severe
4 Very Severe
5 Worst Possible

Mark the area where the pain occurs with the number which corresponds to the intensity of the pain.

### In general, today I felt:

☐ Good

☐ Fair

☐ Poor

# Today's Conditions and Symptoms

Check the areas which apply and explain your conditions symptoms in the space provided. See the *Symptoms Glossary* to help you describe your conditions.

☐ *Ears / Eyes / Nose*

_____

☐ *Mouth / Throat*

_____

☐ *Head / Neck / Back*

_____

☐ *Shoulders / Arms / Hands*

_____

☐ *Chest / Heart*

_____

☐ *Respiratory System*

_____

☐ *Digestive System*

_____

☐ *Hips / Legs / Feet*

_____

☐ *Male / Female Organs*

_____

☐ *Skin*

_____

☐ *Mood*

_____

☐ *Other*

_____

## Comments

_____
_____
_____
_____

MemoryMinder©

## Today's Diet

In columns A&B, list the nutritional facts you wish to monitor (i.e. fat, calories, sodium, sugar, protein, etc.)

☐ **Breakfast**

| | A | B |
|---|---|---|
| | | |
| | | |
| | | |
| | | |
| | | |
| Breakfast Totals | | |

☐ **Lunch**

| | A | B |
|---|---|---|
| | | |
| | | |
| | | |
| | | |
| | | |
| Lunch Totals | | |

☐ **Dinner**

| | A | B |
|---|---|---|
| | | |
| | | |
| | | |
| | | |
| | | |
| Dinner Totals | | |

☐ **Snacks**

| | A | B |
|---|---|---|
| | | |
| | | |
| | | |
| Snack Totals | | |

GRAND TOTALS FOR TODAY:

| A | B |
|---|---|
| | |

| | Date | | Day |
|---|---|---|---|

| | AM | PM |
|---|---|---|
| Weight | | |
| Temperature | | |
| Blood Pressure | | |
| Sugar Level | | |
| Hours slept last night | Number of hours: | Sound ☐ Restless ☐ |
| Naps taken today | How many? | Total hours: |

## Today's Weather

☐ Hot      ☐ Sunny      ☐ Damp
☐ Warm     ☐ Cloudy     ☐ Rainy
☐ Cool     ☐ Overcast   ☐ Snowy
☐ Cold     ☐ Foggy      ☐ Windy

## Drugs / Medications

| Qty | | Description | Strength |
|---|---|---|---|
| AM | PM | | |
| | | | |
| | | | |
| | | | |
| | | | |
| | | | |
| | | | |

## Vitamins / Herbs

| Qty | | Description | Strength |
|---|---|---|---|
| AM | PM | | |
| | | | |
| | | | |
| | | | |
| | | | |
| | | | |
| | | | |

MemoryMinder©

## Physical Activity

| Activity | Hours | Mins. |
|---|---|---|
| | | |
| | | |
| | | |

## Pain / Discomfort / Skin Changes

### Scale

1 Mild
2 Moderate
3 Severe
4 Very Severe
5 Worst Possible

Mark the area where the pain occurs with the number which corresponds to the intensity of the pain.

### In general, today I felt:

☐ Good
☐ Fair
☐ Poor

## Today's Conditions and Symptoms

Check the areas which apply and explain your conditions or symptoms in the space provided. See the *Symptoms Glossary* to help you describe your conditions.

☐ *Ears / Eyes / Nose*
_____

☐ *Mouth / Throat*
_____

☐ *Head / Neck / Back*
_____

☐ *Shoulders / Arms / Hands*
_____

☐ *Chest / Heart*
_____

☐ *Respiratory System*
_____

☐ *Digestive System*
_____

☐ *Hips / Legs / Feet*
_____

☐ *Male / Female Organs*
_____

☐ *Skin*
_____

☐ *Mood*
_____

☐ *Other*
_____
_____

## Comments
_____
_____
_____
_____

MemoryMinder©

## Today's Diet

In columns A&B, list the nutritional facts you wish to monitor (i.e. fat, calories, sodium, sugar, protein, etc.)

| ☐ *Breakfast* | A | B |
|---|---|---|
| | | |
| | | |
| | | |
| | | |
| | | |
| Breakfast Totals | | |

| ☐ *Lunch* | | |
|---|---|---|
| | | |
| | | |
| | | |
| | | |
| | | |
| Lunch Totals | | |

| ☐ *Dinner* | | |
|---|---|---|
| | | |
| | | |
| | | |
| | | |
| | | |
| Dinner Totals | | |

| ☐ *Snacks* | | |
|---|---|---|
| | | |
| | | |
| | | |
| Snack Totals | | |

GRAND TOTALS FOR TODAY:

| A | B |
|---|---|
| | |

|  | | AM | PM |
|---|---|---|---|
| Weight | | | |
| Temperature | | | |
| Blood Pressure | | | |
| Sugar Level | | | |
| Hours slept last night | Number of hours: | | Sound ☐ Restless ☐ |
| Naps taken today | How many? | | Total hours: |

_____  _____
Date                      Day

## Today's Weather

☐ Hot      ☐ Sunny      ☐ Damp
☐ Warm    ☐ Cloudy     ☐ Rainy
☐ Cool     ☐ Overcast   ☐ Snowy
☐ Cold     ☐ Foggy      ☐ Windy

## Drugs / Medications

| Qty | | Description | Strength |
|---|---|---|---|
| AM | PM | | |
| | | | |
| | | | |
| | | | |
| | | | |
| | | | |
| | | | |
| | | | |

## Vitamins / Herbs

| Qty | | Description | Strength |
|---|---|---|---|
| AM | PM | | |
| | | | |
| | | | |
| | | | |
| | | | |
| | | | |
| | | | |
| | | | |

MemoryMinder©

## Physical Activity

| Activity | Hours | Mins. |
|---|---|---|
| | | |
| | | |
| | | |
| | | |

## Pain / Discomfort / Skin Changes

### Scale

1 Mild
2 Moderate
3 Severe
4 Very Severe
5 Worst Possible

Mark the area where the pain occurs with the number which corresponds to the intensity of the pain.

### In general, today I felt:

☐ Good
☐ Fair
☐ Poor

## Today's Conditions and Symptoms

Check the areas which apply and explain your conditions or symptoms in the space provided. See the *Symptoms Glossary* to help you describe your conditions.

☐ *Ears / Eyes / Nose*

☐ *Mouth / Throat*

☐ *Head / Neck / Back*

☐ *Shoulders / Arms / Hands*

☐ *Chest / Heart*

☐ *Respiratory System*

☐ *Digestive System*

☐ *Hips / Legs / Feet*

☐ *Male / Female Organs*

☐ *Skin*

☐ *Mood*

☐ *Other*

## Comments

## Today's Diet

In columns A&B, list the nutritional facts you wish to monitor (i.e. fat, calories, sodium, sugar, protein, etc.)

☐ **Breakfast**

| | A | B |
|---|---|---|
| | | |
| | | |
| | | |
| | | |
| | | |
| Breakfast Totals | | |

☐ **Lunch**

| | A | B |
|---|---|---|
| | | |
| | | |
| | | |
| | | |
| | | |
| Lunch Totals | | |

☐ **Dinner**

| | A | B |
|---|---|---|
| | | |
| | | |
| | | |
| | | |
| | | |
| Dinner Totals | | |

☐ **Snacks**

| | A | B |
|---|---|---|
| | | |
| | | |
| | | |
| Snack Totals | | |

GRAND TOTALS FOR TODAY:

| A | B |
|---|---|
| | |

MemoryMinder©

_____ _____
Date            Day

|                       | AM | PM |
|-----------------------|----|----|
| Weight                |    |    |
| Temperature           |    |    |
| Blood Pressure        |    |    |
| Sugar Level           |    |    |
| Hours slept last night | Number of hours: | Sound ☐ Restless ☐ |
| Naps taken today      | How many? | Total hours: |

## Today's Weather

☐ Hot        ☐ Sunny       ☐ Damp
☐ Warm       ☐ Cloudy      ☐ Rainy
☐ Cool       ☐ Overcast    ☐ Snowy
☐ Cold       ☐ Foggy       ☐ Windy

## Drugs / Medications

| Qty | | Description | Strength |
|-----|-----|-------------|----------|
| AM | PM | | |
| | | | |
| | | | |
| | | | |
| | | | |
| | | | |
| | | | |

## Vitamins / Herbs

| Qty | | Description | Strength |
|-----|-----|-------------|----------|
| AM | PM | | |
| | | | |
| | | | |
| | | | |
| | | | |
| | | | |
| | | | |

MemoryMinder©

## Physical Activity

| Activity | Hours | Mins. |
|----------|-------|-------|
| | | |
| | | |
| | | |
| | | |

## Pain / Discomfort / Skin Changes

### Scale

1 Mild
2 Moderate
3 Severe
4 Very Severe
5 Worst Possible

Mark the area where the pain occurs with the number which corresponds to the intensity of the pain.

### In general, today I felt:

☐ Good
☐ Fair
☐ Poor

# Today's Conditions and Symptoms

Check the areas which apply and explain your conditions
or symptoms in the space provided. See the *Symptoms
Glossary* to help you describe your conditions.

☐ *Ears / Eyes / Nose*

_____

☐ *Mouth / Throat*

_____

☐ *Head / Neck / Back*

_____

☐ *Shoulders / Arms / Hands*

_____

☐ *Chest / Heart*

_____

☐ *Respiratory System*

_____

☐ *Digestive System*

_____

☐ *Hips / Legs / Feet*

_____

☐ *Male / Female Organs*

_____

☐ *Skin*

_____

☐ *Mood*

_____

☐ *Other*

_____

_____

## Comments

_____
_____
_____
_____

MemoryMinder©

## Today's Diet

In columns A&B, list the nutritional
facts you wish to monitor (i.e. fat,
calories, sodium, sugar, protein, etc.)

☐ **Breakfast**

| | A | B |
|---|---|---|
| | | |
| | | |
| | | |
| | | |
| | | |
| Breakfast Totals | | |

☐ **Lunch**

| | | |
|---|---|---|
| | | |
| | | |
| | | |
| | | |
| | | |
| Lunch Totals | | |

☐ **Dinner**

| | | |
|---|---|---|
| | | |
| | | |
| | | |
| | | |
| | | |
| Dinner Totals | | |

☐ **Snacks**

| | | |
|---|---|---|
| | | |
| | | |
| | | |
| Snack Totals | | |

GRAND TOTALS FOR TODAY:

| A | B |
|---|---|
| | |

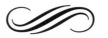

# Additional
# Health Records

# ~Personal Medical History~

If you record your medical history below, this record will be a handy reference when visiting your physician, filling out new-patient questionaires, or for your own general information.

| Childhood Illnesses and Diseases | Date |
|---|---|
|  |  |
|  |  |
|  |  |
|  |  |

| Adult Illnesses and Diseases | Date |
|---|---|
|  |  |
|  |  |
|  |  |
|  |  |

| Serious Injuries | Date |
|---|---|
|  |  |
|  |  |
|  |  |

| Surgeries | Date |
|---|---|
|  |  |
|  |  |
|  |  |
|  |  |

| Vaccinations, Etc. | Date | Date | Date | Date |
|---|---|---|---|---|
| Flu Shot | | | | |
| Pneumonia Shot | | | | |
| Polio | | | | |
| Tetanus | | | | |
| | | | | |
| | | | | |
| | | | | |
| | | | | |

### Blood Type _____

| | | | | | |
|---|---|---|---|---|---|
| **Blood Donation Dates** | | | | | |
| **Blood Transfusion Dates** | | | | | |

| Allergies | Reactions |
|---|---|
| | |
| | |
| | |
| | |
| | |

### Other Information

# ~Medical Tests~

| Type of Test | Date | Result | Date | Result | Date | Result |
|---|---|---|---|---|---|---|
| Biopsy | | | | | | |
| Blood Count | | | | | | |
| Blood Glucose | | | | | | |
| CAT Scan | | | | | | |
| Chest X-ray | | | | | | |
| Cholesterol Count | | | | | | |
| Complete Physical | | | | | | |
| Dental X-ray | | | | | | |
| EKG | | | | | | |
| Glaucoma Screening | | | | | | |
| Hearing | | | | | | |
| Hemoglobin $A_{1C}$ | | | | | | |
| MRI | | | | | | |
| Mammogram | | | | | | |
| PAP Smear | | | | | | |
| Pregnancy | | | | | | |
| Rubella | | | | | | |
| Stool (Colon) Screen | | | | | | |
| TB | | | | | | |
| Thyroid | | | | | | |
| Urinalysis | | | | | | |
| Vision | | | | | | |
| | | | | | | |
| | | | | | | |
| | | | | | | |
| | | | | | | |
| | | | | | | |
| | | | | | | |

# ~Insurance & Pharmacies~

## Insurance Carriers

Company

Policy Number

Address

Phone/fax

Company

Policy Number

Address

Phone/fax

Company

Policy Number

Address

Phone/fax

## Pharmacies

Name

Address

Phone/fax

Name

Address

Phone/fax

Name

Address

Phone/fax

Name

Address

Phone/fax

Name

Address

Phone/fax

# ~Health-Care Providers~

## Doctors, Nurses, Clinics, Hospitals, etc.

Name

Address

City, Zip

Phone/fax

Name

Address

City, Zip

Phone/fax

Name

Address

City, Zip

Phone/fax

Name

Address

City, Zip

Phone/fax

Name

Address

City, Zip

Phone/fax

Name

Address

City, Zip

Phone/fax

Name

Address

City, Zip

Phone/fax

# ~Purchase Record~

| Date | Item / Description | Qty. | Price | Store |
|------|--------------------|------|-------|-------|
| | **Vitamins, medications, supplies, etc.** | | | |
| | | | | |
| | | | | |
| | | | | |
| | | | | |
| | | | | |
| | | | | |
| | | | | |
| | | | | |
| | | | | |
| | | | | |
| | | | | |
| | | | | |
| | | | | |
| | | | | |
| | | | | |
| | | | | |
| | | | | |
| | | | | |
| | | | | |
| | | | | |
| | | | | |
| | | | | |
| | | | | |
| | | | | |
| | | | | |
| | | | | |
| | | | | |
| | | | | |
| | | | | |
| | | | | |
| | | | | |
| | | | | |
| | | | | |
| | | | | |
| | | | | |

# ~Notes & Questions~

Suggestions: List questions that arise between health-care visits.
Record answers and advice including date and name of doctor or advice-giver.

| Date | |
|------|--|
| | |
| | |
| | |
| | |
| | |
| | |
| | |
| | |
| | |
| | |
| | |
| | |
| | |
| | |
| | |
| | |
| | |
| | |
| | |
| | |
| | |
| | |
| | |
| | |
| | |

# ~Notes and Questions~

| Date | |
|------|---|
| | |

# ~Notes and Questions~

| Date | |
|------|--|
|      |  |
|      |  |
|      |  |
|      |  |
|      |  |
|      |  |
|      |  |
|      |  |
|      |  |
|      |  |
|      |  |
|      |  |
|      |  |
|      |  |
|      |  |
|      |  |
|      |  |
|      |  |
|      |  |
|      |  |
|      |  |
|      |  |
|      |  |
|      |  |
|      |  |
|      |  |
|      |  |
|      |  |
|      |  |
|      |  |
|      |  |

# ~Notes and Questions~

| Date | |
|------|---|
|  |  |
|  |  |
|  |  |
|  |  |
|  |  |
|  |  |
|  |  |
|  |  |
|  |  |
|  |  |
|  |  |
|  |  |
|  |  |
|  |  |
|  |  |
|  |  |
|  |  |
|  |  |
|  |  |
|  |  |
|  |  |
|  |  |
|  |  |
|  |  |
|  |  |
|  |  |
|  |  |
|  |  |
|  |  |
|  |  |

# 2005

## January
| S | M | T | W | T | F | S |
|---|---|---|---|---|---|---|
|  |  |  |  |  |  | 1 |
| 2 | 3 | 4 | 5 | 6 | 7 | 8 |
| 9 | 10 | 11 | 12 | 13 | 14 | 15 |
| 16 | 17 | 18 | 19 | 20 | 21 | 22 |
| 23 | 24 | 25 | 26 | 27 | 28 | 29 |
| 30 | 31 |  |  |  |  |  |

## February
| S | M | T | W | T | F | S |
|---|---|---|---|---|---|---|
|  |  | 1 | 2 | 3 | 4 | 5 |
| 6 | 7 | 8 | 9 | 10 | 11 | 12 |
| 13 | 14 | 15 | 16 | 17 | 18 | 19 |
| 20 | 21 | 22 | 23 | 24 | 25 | 26 |
| 27 | 28 |  |  |  |  |  |

## March
| S | M | T | W | T | F | S |
|---|---|---|---|---|---|---|
|  |  | 1 | 2 | 3 | 4 | 5 |
| 6 | 7 | 8 | 9 | 10 | 11 | 12 |
| 13 | 14 | 15 | 16 | 17 | 18 | 19 |
| 20 | 21 | 22 | 23 | 24 | 25 | 26 |
| 27 | 28 | 29 | 30 | 31 |  |  |

## April
| S | M | T | W | T | F | S |
|---|---|---|---|---|---|---|
|  |  |  |  |  | 1 | 2 |
| 3 | 4 | 5 | 6 | 7 | 8 | 9 |
| 10 | 11 | 12 | 13 | 14 | 15 | 16 |
| 17 | 18 | 19 | 20 | 21 | 22 | 23 |
| 24 | 25 | 26 | 27 | 28 | 29 | 30 |

## May
| S | M | T | W | T | F | S |
|---|---|---|---|---|---|---|
| 1 | 2 | 3 | 4 | 5 | 6 | 7 |
| 8 | 9 | 10 | 11 | 12 | 13 | 14 |
| 15 | 16 | 17 | 18 | 19 | 20 | 21 |
| 22 | 23 | 24 | 25 | 26 | 27 | 28 |
| 29 | 30 | 31 |  |  |  |  |

## June
| S | M | T | W | T | F | S |
|---|---|---|---|---|---|---|
|  |  |  | 1 | 2 | 3 | 4 |
| 5 | 6 | 7 | 8 | 9 | 10 | 11 |
| 12 | 13 | 14 | 15 | 16 | 17 | 18 |
| 19 | 20 | 21 | 22 | 23 | 24 | 25 |
| 26 | 27 | 28 | 29 | 30 |  |  |

## July
| S | M | T | W | T | F | S |
|---|---|---|---|---|---|---|
|  |  |  |  |  | 1 | 2 |
| 3 | 4 | 5 | 6 | 7 | 8 | 9 |
| 10 | 11 | 12 | 13 | 14 | 15 | 16 |
| 17 | 18 | 19 | 20 | 21 | 22 | 23 |
| 24 | 25 | 26 | 27 | 28 | 29 | 30 |
| 31 |  |  |  |  |  |  |

## August
| S | M | T | W | T | F | S |
|---|---|---|---|---|---|---|
|  | 1 | 2 | 3 | 4 | 5 | 6 |
| 7 | 8 | 9 | 10 | 11 | 12 | 13 |
| 14 | 15 | 16 | 17 | 18 | 19 | 20 |
| 21 | 22 | 23 | 24 | 25 | 26 | 27 |
| 28 | 29 | 30 | 31 |  |  |  |

## September
| S | M | T | W | T | F | S |
|---|---|---|---|---|---|---|
|  |  |  |  | 1 | 2 | 3 |
| 4 | 5 | 6 | 7 | 8 | 9 | 10 |
| 11 | 12 | 13 | 14 | 15 | 16 | 17 |
| 18 | 19 | 20 | 21 | 22 | 23 | 24 |
| 25 | 26 | 27 | 28 | 29 | 30 |  |

## October
| S | M | T | W | T | F | S |
|---|---|---|---|---|---|---|
|  |  |  |  |  |  | 1 |
| 2 | 3 | 4 | 5 | 6 | 7 | 8 |
| 9 | 10 | 11 | 12 | 13 | 14 | 15 |
| 16 | 17 | 18 | 19 | 20 | 21 | 22 |
| 23 | 24 | 25 | 26 | 27 | 28 | 29 |
| 30 | 31 |  |  |  |  |  |

## November
| S | M | T | W | T | F | S |
|---|---|---|---|---|---|---|
|  |  | 1 | 2 | 3 | 4 | 5 |
| 6 | 7 | 8 | 9 | 10 | 11 | 12 |
| 13 | 14 | 15 | 16 | 17 | 18 | 19 |
| 20 | 21 | 22 | 23 | 24 | 25 | 26 |
| 27 | 28 | 29 | 30 |  |  |  |

## December
| S | M | T | W | T | F | S |
|---|---|---|---|---|---|---|
|  |  |  |  | 1 | 2 | 3 |
| 4 | 5 | 6 | 7 | 8 | 9 | 10 |
| 11 | 12 | 13 | 14 | 15 | 16 | 17 |
| 18 | 19 | 20 | 21 | 22 | 23 | 24 |
| 25 | 26 | 27 | 28 | 29 | 30 | 31 |

MemoryMinder Journals, Inc.©

# 2006

## January
| S | M | T | W | T | F | S |
|---|---|---|---|---|---|---|
| 1 | 2 | 3 | 4 | 5 | 6 | 7 |
| 8 | 9 | 10 | 11 | 12 | 13 | 14 |
| 15 | 16 | 17 | 18 | 19 | 20 | 21 |
| 22 | 23 | 24 | 25 | 26 | 27 | 28 |
| 29 | 30 | 31 |  |  |  |  |

## February
| S | M | T | W | T | F | S |
|---|---|---|---|---|---|---|
|  |  |  | 1 | 2 | 3 | 4 |
| 5 | 6 | 7 | 8 | 9 | 10 | 11 |
| 12 | 13 | 14 | 15 | 16 | 17 | 18 |
| 19 | 20 | 21 | 22 | 23 | 24 | 25 |
| 26 | 27 | 28 |  |  |  |  |

## March
| S | M | T | W | T | F | S |
|---|---|---|---|---|---|---|
|  |  |  | 1 | 2 | 3 | 4 |
| 5 | 6 | 7 | 8 | 9 | 10 | 11 |
| 12 | 13 | 14 | 15 | 16 | 17 | 18 |
| 19 | 20 | 21 | 22 | 23 | 24 | 25 |
| 26 | 27 | 28 | 29 | 30 | 31 |  |

## April
| S | M | T | W | T | F | S |
|---|---|---|---|---|---|---|
|  |  |  |  |  |  | 1 |
| 2 | 3 | 4 | 5 | 6 | 7 | 8 |
| 9 | 10 | 11 | 12 | 13 | 14 | 15 |
| 16 | 17 | 18 | 19 | 20 | 21 | 22 |
| 23 | 24 | 25 | 26 | 27 | 28 | 29 |
| 30 |  |  |  |  |  |  |

## May
| S | M | T | W | T | F | S |
|---|---|---|---|---|---|---|
|  | 1 | 2 | 3 | 4 | 5 | 6 |
| 7 | 8 | 9 | 10 | 11 | 12 | 13 |
| 14 | 15 | 16 | 17 | 18 | 19 | 20 |
| 21 | 22 | 23 | 24 | 25 | 26 | 27 |
| 28 | 29 | 30 | 31 |  |  |  |

## June
| S | M | T | W | T | F | S |
|---|---|---|---|---|---|---|
|  |  |  |  | 1 | 2 | 3 |
| 4 | 5 | 6 | 7 | 8 | 9 | 10 |
| 11 | 12 | 13 | 14 | 15 | 16 | 17 |
| 18 | 19 | 20 | 21 | 22 | 23 | 24 |
| 25 | 26 | 27 | 28 | 29 | 30 |  |

## July
| S | M | T | W | T | F | S |
|---|---|---|---|---|---|---|
|  |  |  |  |  |  | 1 |
| 2 | 3 | 4 | 5 | 6 | 7 | 8 |
| 9 | 10 | 11 | 12 | 13 | 14 | 15 |
| 16 | 17 | 18 | 19 | 20 | 21 | 22 |
| 23 | 24 | 25 | 26 | 27 | 28 | 29 |
| 30 | 31 |  |  |  |  |  |

## August
| S | M | T | W | T | F | S |
|---|---|---|---|---|---|---|
|  |  | 1 | 2 | 3 | 4 | 5 |
| 6 | 7 | 8 | 9 | 10 | 11 | 12 |
| 13 | 14 | 15 | 16 | 17 | 18 | 19 |
| 20 | 21 | 22 | 23 | 24 | 25 | 26 |
| 27 | 28 | 29 | 30 | 31 |  |  |

## September
| S | M | T | W | T | F | S |
|---|---|---|---|---|---|---|
|  |  |  |  |  | 1 | 2 |
| 3 | 4 | 5 | 6 | 7 | 8 | 9 |
| 10 | 11 | 12 | 13 | 14 | 15 | 16 |
| 17 | 18 | 19 | 20 | 21 | 22 | 23 |
| 24 | 25 | 26 | 27 | 28 | 29 | 30 |

## October
| S | M | T | W | T | F | S |
|---|---|---|---|---|---|---|
| 1 | 2 | 3 | 4 | 5 | 6 | 7 |
| 8 | 9 | 10 | 11 | 12 | 13 | 14 |
| 15 | 16 | 17 | 18 | 19 | 20 | 21 |
| 22 | 23 | 24 | 25 | 26 | 27 | 28 |
| 29 | 30 | 31 |  |  |  |  |

## November
| S | M | T | W | T | F | S |
|---|---|---|---|---|---|---|
|  |  |  | 1 | 2 | 3 | 4 |
| 5 | 6 | 7 | 8 | 9 | 10 | 11 |
| 12 | 13 | 14 | 15 | 16 | 17 | 18 |
| 19 | 20 | 21 | 22 | 23 | 24 | 25 |
| 26 | 27 | 28 | 29 | 30 |  |  |

## December
| S | M | T | W | T | F | S |
|---|---|---|---|---|---|---|
|  |  |  |  |  | 1 | 2 |
| 3 | 4 | 5 | 6 | 7 | 8 | 9 |
| 10 | 11 | 12 | 13 | 14 | 15 | 16 |
| 17 | 18 | 19 | 20 | 21 | 22 | 23 |
| 24 | 25 | 26 | 27 | 28 | 29 | 30 |
| 31 |  |  |  |  |  |  |

## 2007

### January
| S | M | T | W | T | F | S |
|---|---|---|---|---|---|---|
|  | 1 | 2 | 3 | 4 | 5 | 6 |
| 7 | 8 | 9 | 10 | 11 | 12 | 13 |
| 14 | 15 | 16 | 17 | 18 | 19 | 20 |
| 21 | 22 | 23 | 24 | 25 | 26 | 27 |
| 28 | 29 | 30 | 31 |  |  |  |

### February
| S | M | T | W | T | F | S |
|---|---|---|---|---|---|---|
|  |  |  |  | 1 | 2 | 3 |
| 4 | 5 | 6 | 7 | 8 | 9 | 10 |
| 11 | 12 | 13 | 14 | 15 | 16 | 17 |
| 18 | 19 | 20 | 21 | 22 | 23 | 24 |
| 25 | 26 | 27 | 28 |  |  |  |

### March
| S | M | T | W | T | F | S |
|---|---|---|---|---|---|---|
|  |  |  |  | 1 | 2 | 3 |
| 4 | 5 | 6 | 7 | 8 | 9 | 10 |
| 11 | 12 | 13 | 14 | 15 | 16 | 17 |
| 18 | 19 | 20 | 21 | 22 | 23 | 24 |
| 25 | 26 | 27 | 28 | 29 | 30 | 31 |

### April
| S | M | T | W | T | F | S |
|---|---|---|---|---|---|---|
| 1 | 2 | 3 | 4 | 5 | 6 | 7 |
| 8 | 9 | 10 | 11 | 12 | 13 | 14 |
| 15 | 16 | 17 | 18 | 19 | 20 | 21 |
| 22 | 23 | 24 | 25 | 26 | 27 | 28 |
| 29 | 30 |  |  |  |  |  |

### May
| S | M | T | W | T | F | S |
|---|---|---|---|---|---|---|
|  |  | 1 | 2 | 3 | 4 | 5 |
| 6 | 7 | 8 | 9 | 10 | 11 | 12 |
| 13 | 14 | 15 | 16 | 17 | 18 | 19 |
| 20 | 21 | 22 | 23 | 24 | 25 | 26 |
| 27 | 28 | 29 | 30 | 31 |  |  |

### June
| S | M | T | W | T | F | S |
|---|---|---|---|---|---|---|
|  |  |  |  |  | 1 | 2 |
| 3 | 4 | 5 | 6 | 7 | 8 | 9 |
| 10 | 11 | 12 | 13 | 14 | 15 | 16 |
| 17 | 18 | 19 | 20 | 21 | 22 | 23 |
| 24 | 25 | 26 | 27 | 28 | 29 | 30 |

### July
| S | M | T | W | T | F | S |
|---|---|---|---|---|---|---|
| 1 | 2 | 3 | 4 | 5 | 6 | 7 |
| 8 | 9 | 10 | 11 | 12 | 13 | 14 |
| 15 | 16 | 17 | 18 | 19 | 20 | 21 |
| 22 | 23 | 24 | 25 | 26 | 27 | 28 |
| 29 | 30 | 31 |  |  |  |  |

### August
| S | M | T | W | T | F | S |
|---|---|---|---|---|---|---|
|  |  |  | 1 | 2 | 3 | 4 |
| 5 | 6 | 7 | 8 | 9 | 10 | 11 |
| 12 | 13 | 14 | 15 | 16 | 17 | 18 |
| 19 | 20 | 21 | 22 | 23 | 24 | 25 |
| 26 | 27 | 28 | 29 | 30 | 31 |  |

### September
| S | M | T | W | T | F | S |
|---|---|---|---|---|---|---|
|  |  |  |  |  |  | 1 |
| 2 | 3 | 4 | 5 | 6 | 7 | 8 |
| 9 | 10 | 11 | 12 | 13 | 14 | 15 |
| 16 | 17 | 18 | 19 | 20 | 21 | 22 |
| 23 | 24 | 25 | 26 | 27 | 28 | 29 |
| 30 |  |  |  |  |  |  |

### October
| S | M | T | W | T | F | S |
|---|---|---|---|---|---|---|
|  | 1 | 2 | 3 | 4 | 5 | 6 |
| 7 | 8 | 9 | 10 | 11 | 12 | 13 |
| 14 | 15 | 16 | 17 | 18 | 19 | 20 |
| 21 | 22 | 23 | 24 | 25 | 26 | 27 |
| 28 | 29 | 30 | 31 |  |  |  |

### November
| S | M | T | W | T | F | S |
|---|---|---|---|---|---|---|
|  |  |  |  | 1 | 2 | 3 |
| 4 | 5 | 6 | 7 | 8 | 9 | 10 |
| 11 | 12 | 13 | 14 | 15 | 16 | 17 |
| 18 | 19 | 20 | 21 | 22 | 23 | 24 |
| 25 | 26 | 27 | 28 | 29 | 30 |  |

### December
| S | M | T | W | T | F | S |
|---|---|---|---|---|---|---|
|  |  |  |  |  |  | 1 |
| 2 | 3 | 4 | 5 | 6 | 7 | 8 |
| 9 | 10 | 11 | 12 | 13 | 14 | 15 |
| 16 | 17 | 18 | 19 | 20 | 21 | 22 |
| 23 | 24 | 25 | 26 | 27 | 28 | 29 |
| 30 | 31 |  |  |  |  |  |

MemoryMinder Journals, Inc.©

## 2008

### January
| S | M | T | W | T | F | S |
|---|---|---|---|---|---|---|
|  |  | 1 | 2 | 3 | 4 | 5 |
| 6 | 7 | 8 | 9 | 10 | 11 | 12 |
| 13 | 14 | 15 | 16 | 17 | 18 | 19 |
| 20 | 21 | 22 | 23 | 24 | 25 | 26 |
| 27 | 28 | 29 | 30 | 31 |  |  |

### February
| S | M | T | W | T | F | S |
|---|---|---|---|---|---|---|
|  |  |  |  |  | 1 | 2 |
| 3 | 4 | 5 | 6 | 7 | 8 | 9 |
| 10 | 11 | 12 | 13 | 14 | 15 | 16 |
| 17 | 18 | 19 | 20 | 21 | 22 | 23 |
| 24 | 25 | 26 | 27 | 28 | 29 |  |

### March
| S | M | T | W | T | F | S |
|---|---|---|---|---|---|---|
|  |  |  |  |  |  | 1 |
| 2 | 3 | 4 | 5 | 6 | 7 | 8 |
| 9 | 10 | 11 | 12 | 13 | 14 | 15 |
| 16 | 17 | 18 | 19 | 20 | 21 | 22 |
| 23 | 24 | 25 | 26 | 27 | 28 | 29 |
| 30 | 31 |  |  |  |  |  |

### April
| S | M | T | W | T | F | S |
|---|---|---|---|---|---|---|
|  |  | 1 | 2 | 3 | 4 | 5 |
| 6 | 7 | 8 | 9 | 10 | 11 | 12 |
| 13 | 14 | 15 | 16 | 17 | 18 | 19 |
| 20 | 21 | 22 | 23 | 24 | 25 | 26 |
| 27 | 28 | 29 | 30 |  |  |  |

### May
| S | M | T | W | T | F | S |
|---|---|---|---|---|---|---|
|  |  |  |  | 1 | 2 | 3 |
| 4 | 5 | 6 | 7 | 8 | 9 | 10 |
| 11 | 12 | 13 | 14 | 15 | 16 | 17 |
| 18 | 19 | 20 | 21 | 22 | 23 | 24 |
| 25 | 26 | 27 | 28 | 29 | 30 | 31 |

### June
| S | M | T | W | T | F | S |
|---|---|---|---|---|---|---|
| 1 | 2 | 3 | 4 | 5 | 6 | 7 |
| 8 | 9 | 10 | 11 | 12 | 13 | 14 |
| 15 | 16 | 17 | 18 | 19 | 20 | 21 |
| 22 | 23 | 24 | 25 | 26 | 27 | 28 |
| 29 | 30 |  |  |  |  |  |

### July
| S | M | T | W | T | F | S |
|---|---|---|---|---|---|---|
|  |  | 1 | 2 | 3 | 4 | 5 |
| 6 | 7 | 8 | 9 | 10 | 11 | 12 |
| 13 | 14 | 15 | 16 | 17 | 18 | 19 |
| 20 | 21 | 22 | 23 | 24 | 25 | 26 |
| 27 | 28 | 29 | 30 | 31 |  |  |

### August
| S | M | T | W | T | F | S |
|---|---|---|---|---|---|---|
|  |  |  |  |  | 1 | 2 |
| 3 | 4 | 5 | 6 | 7 | 8 | 9 |
| 10 | 11 | 12 | 13 | 14 | 15 | 16 |
| 17 | 18 | 19 | 20 | 21 | 22 | 23 |
| 24 | 25 | 26 | 27 | 28 | 29 | 30 |
| 31 |  |  |  |  |  |  |

### September
| S | M | T | W | T | F | S |
|---|---|---|---|---|---|---|
|  | 1 | 2 | 3 | 4 | 5 | 6 |
| 7 | 8 | 9 | 10 | 11 | 12 | 13 |
| 14 | 15 | 16 | 17 | 18 | 19 | 20 |
| 21 | 22 | 23 | 24 | 25 | 26 | 27 |
| 28 | 29 | 30 |  |  |  |  |

### October
| S | M | T | W | T | F | S |
|---|---|---|---|---|---|---|
|  |  |  | 1 | 2 | 3 | 4 |
| 5 | 6 | 7 | 8 | 9 | 10 | 11 |
| 12 | 13 | 14 | 15 | 16 | 17 | 18 |
| 19 | 20 | 21 | 22 | 23 | 24 | 25 |
| 26 | 27 | 28 | 29 | 30 | 31 |  |

### November
| S | M | T | W | T | F | S |
|---|---|---|---|---|---|---|
|  |  |  |  |  |  | 1 |
| 2 | 3 | 4 | 5 | 6 | 7 | 8 |
| 9 | 10 | 11 | 12 | 13 | 14 | 15 |
| 16 | 17 | 18 | 19 | 20 | 21 | 22 |
| 23 | 24 | 25 | 26 | 27 | 28 | 29 |
| 30 |  |  |  |  |  |  |

### December
| S | M | T | W | T | F | S |
|---|---|---|---|---|---|---|
|  | 1 | 2 | 3 | 4 | 5 | 6 |
| 7 | 8 | 9 | 10 | 11 | 12 | 13 |
| 14 | 15 | 16 | 17 | 18 | 19 | 20 |
| 21 | 22 | 23 | 24 | 25 | 26 | 27 |
| 28 | 29 | 30 | 31 |  |  |  |

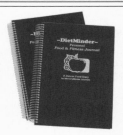
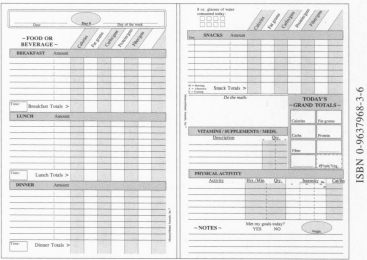

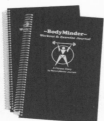

# ~BodyMinder~

## Workout & Exercise Journal

### A Physical Fitness Diary

Whether you workout regularly or are just beginning, the BodyMinder can help you stay on track and keep you motivated...whatever your goal.

Designed originally for gyms and health clubs, this handy journal has become a favorite with fitness buffs *wherever* they work out...at the gym, at home, or anywhere their activities take them.

The BodyMinder works for *all* types of exercise, from weight training to aerobics to sporting activities. Even housework can be recorded. With the BodyMinder you'll soon see your goals become reality!

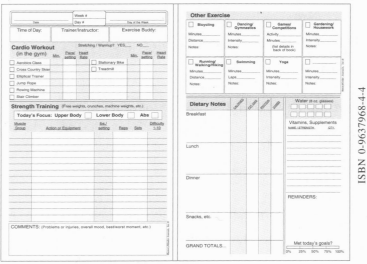

*BodyMinder Daily Pages*

### In the **BodyMinder** you can record your:

- Starting statistics • Goals • Weekly plans • Progress • Games • Expenses
- Daily workout details such as...reps, sets, time spent, equipment, settings
- More daily details including...other exercise, meals, food counts, vitamins, etc.

---

- All journals feature durable leatherette covers in choice of colors
- Convenient size for home or travel (8.5" X 6") • Spiral-binding for ease of writing • 224 pages for up to three months of daily records
- Handy reference calendars • Vinyl pocket for appointment cards, prescriptions, receipts, schedules, recipes, etc.

*See next page for ordering information* *

## To order additional Journals...

Mail this order form with your check or money order to:
**MemoryMinder Journals**
**PO Box 23108 • Eugene, OR 97402-0425**
*(Please allow 1-2 weeks for delivery)*
**For Visa/Mastercard orders call 1(800) 888-3392**
For more information
or quotes on large quantities,
please call us or visit our website.
*www.memoryminder.com*

**\*\*SAVE!\*\* When you order more than one, deduct $2 per journal!**

---

### MemoryMinder *Personal Health Journal*

Color and Quantity:

Red_____ Navy_____ @ $14.95 each = $_____

### DietMinder *Personal Food & Fitness Journal*

Color and Quantity:

Plum_____ Forest Green_____ @ $14.95 each = $_____

### BodyMinder *Workout & Exercise Journal*

Color and Quantity:

Black_____ Burgundy_____ @ $14.95 each = $_____

**\*Discount**...$2 off each book when ordering 2 or more: (minus- $_____

**Subtotal** $_____

**Shipping/Handling**: add $3.95 for the first book = $____**3.95**____

...plus $1.00 for each additional book = $_____

**Total** (payment enclosed) = $

I first learned about *MemoryMinder Journals* from:

☐ Magazine ☐ Bookstore ☐ Friend
☐ Internet ☐ Health Store ☐ Other _____

Name_____

Company/organization_____

Mailing Address_____

City_____St_____Zip_____

ISBN 0-9637968-0-1